How to Parent Adult Children

Dealing With Adult Children – How to Communicate, Navigate Transition, Resolve Conflicts, and Set Healthy Boundaries When Parenting Adult Children (A Secular Approach)

Belinda Sparks

eBook ISBN: 978-981-18-9534-0
Paperback ISBN: 978-981-18-9535-7

Table of Contents

Introduction:

Welcome to the Next Chapter

Welcome to a journey that many of us embark upon with love, hope, and a little trepidation—the path of parenting our adult children. I'm Belinda, a mother of two wonderful adults, a son and a daughter, and I want to assure you that I have and continue to travel this sometimes challenging, always evolving, but ultimately rewarding road.

This book is here to offer a guide through the intricate maze of parenting your grown-up children in a world vastly different from the one in which we grew up. It's a world where communication, boundaries, and relationships take on new dimensions, but with the right approach, it's a world where we can thrive as parents and nurture strong connections with our adult offspring.

As parents, we often prepare meticulously for the early years of our children's lives. We read books on pregnancy, childbirth, and child-rearing, attend parenting classes, and seek advice from experts and experienced parents. But what about the next chapter? What about the phase when our children have grown into adults with their own dreams, desires, and challenges? When they pack up and leave our nest, ready to fly free. It's a phase often overlooked, and it's precisely this journey that we'll explore together in the pages of this book.

Throughout the following chapters, we'll explore various aspects of parenting adult children, offering practical advice and strategies to help you navigate this new terrain. We'll discuss topics such as understanding love languages, effective communication, transitioning roles, reconnecting with estranged adult children, setting and respecting boundaries, self-care, and even managing when your adult child decides to move back home, and so much more.

I believe we want the best for our adult children, and with the right guidance and support, we can not only maintain but also enhance our relationships with them. This book aims to provide you with a sense of community, a reassuring hand to hold, and the tools you need to foster strong, healthy, and fulfilling relationships with your adult children.

I'll share real-life examples, a few case studies, and personal stories to illustrate the principles and strategies discussed in these pages. We'll also draw upon expert opinions and research-backed information every now and then to provide you with a well-rounded perspective.

Remember, the relationship you have with your adult children will not mirror the one you had with your own parents, and that's okay. We come from a generation that left home much earlier, so our parents rarely, if ever, had discussions about our emotional state or finances once we were out the door. The world is constantly changing, and so should our approach to parenting. The goal is not to cling to the past but to adapt and grow as our children do.

I want you to approach this journey with hope, knowing that positive change is possible. Together, we'll explore ways to improve your relationship with your adult children, strengthen your bonds, and embrace the joys and challenges that come with this new phase of parenting.

Your adult children are no longer children, but they will always be your wee ones, and your love and support are still as vital as ever. Let's begin this exploration of parenting our adult children with open hearts, open minds, and a commitment to building stronger, more fulfilling relationships.

With warmth and understanding,

Belinda

Chapter 1:

Myers-Briggs Type Indicator-Understanding Your Adult Child's Personality Type

As parents, we all know the profound truth that our children are not mere extensions of ourselves; they are unique individuals with their own dreams, desires, and, yes, quirks. It's a reality we've come to accept, and as we navigate the transition into their adulthood, it's important to embrace this with open arms and open hearts.

One fascinating way to better understand your adult child is by exploring the world of Myers-Briggs Type Indicator (MBTI) personality types. The MBTI is an assessment tool that helps us understand our strengths, weaknesses, and what makes us unique. It's even utilized in certain job application processes to assist employers in determining if a candidate would be a good fit for their company culture and team dynamics. Therefore, MBTI has real-life applications and proven usefulness. Similarly, knowing your child's MBTI personality can aid you in adapting your parenting and communication approach (***Myers-Briggs Overview*, 2023**).

In the pages ahead, I will break down the various personality types outlined by MBTI. My aim is not to put our adult children into boxes or label them, but to offer insights that can enhance your understanding and communication with them. Whether your child is an introvert or an extrovert, a thinker or a feeler, they are still the same beloved person you've known since birth. Understanding their personality type will help you foster a deeper, more meaningful connection and build bridges of communication.

The Personality Types

Once you take the MBTI test, the tool categorizes personalities into 16 distinct types based on four preference pairs: Extraversion (E) or Introversion (I), Sensing (S) or Intuition (N), Thinking (T) or Feeling (F), and Judging (J) or Perceiving (P). Let's break down what each of these preferences means (***Personality Types*, 2023**):

- **Extraversion (E) or Introversion (I):** This is about how your child directs and receives energy. Extraverts are outgoing, sociable, and energized by social interactions, while Introverts are more reserved and need downtime to recharge.

- **Sensing (S) or Intuition (N):** This pair relates to how they take in information. Sensors rely on tangible, concrete details, while Intuitives are more focused on the big picture, patterns, and possibilities.

- **Thinking (T) or Feeling (F):** It's all about how they make decisions. Thinkers prioritize logic and objectivity, while Feelers base decisions on values, emotions, and empathy.

- **Judging (J) or Perceiving (P):** This final pair reflects how they approach the outside world. Judgers prefer structure, organization, and planning, while Perceivers are adaptable, spontaneous, and go with the flow.

When the letters for each of these preferences are combined, 16 distinct personality types form, each consisting of different characteristics unique to that type.

So again, the test will give you a result combining four of these letters in one of the formats discussed further below (***Personality Types*, 2023**).

Introverted, Sensing, Thinking, and Judging (ISTJ)

I'm the type who prefers a calm and composed approach, taking my time to achieve success through thoroughness and reliability. I'm practical, down-to-earth, and have a realistic outlook on life. I'm responsible and make decisions based on logic, staying focused on my goals even in the face of distractions. I find joy in creating order and organization in every aspect of my life, be it work or home. I highly value traditions and loyalty.

Introverted, Sensing, Feeling, and Judging (ISFJ)

I'm the epitome of a great friend and colleague. I'm quiet but super friendly and responsible. You can always count on me to meet my obligations without fail. I'm incredibly thorough, paying attention to every little detail and making sure everything is accurate. Plus, I'm loyal and considerate, always remembering the little things about the people who matter to me. I genuinely care about how others feel and go out of my way to create a harmonious environment, both at work and at home.

Introverted, Intuitive, Feeling, and Judging (INFJ)

I yearn for meaning and connection in ideas, relationships, and material possessions. Understanding what motivates people is important to me, and I possess insight into others. I'm conscientious and deeply committed to my firm values. Developing a clear vision on how to best serve the common good is a priority, and I'm organized and decisive in implementing this vision.

Introverted, Intuitive, Thinking, and Judging (INTJ)

I possess a unique perspective and a strong determination to bring my ideas to life and accomplish my aspirations. I have a keen ability to discern patterns in the world around me and formulate insightful, far-reaching viewpoints. Once I dedicate myself to a task, I excel at organizing and seeing it through to completion. I approach situations with a healthy dose of skepticism and value independence, holding both myself and others to high standards of proficiency and achievement.

Introverted, Sensing, Thinking, and Perceiving (ISTP)

Tolerant and flexible, I'm the type of person who prefers to quietly observe until a problem arises. But when it does, I spring into action, finding quick and workable solutions. I have a knack for analyzing what makes things tick and can easily sift through large amounts of data to pinpoint the core of practical problems. I'm genuinely interested in cause and effect, and I organize facts using logical principles, always valuing efficiency.

Introverted, Sensing, Feeling, and Perceiving (ISFP)

I'm the kind of person who's quiet, friendly, sensitive, and kind. I really enjoy living in the present moment and being aware of what's happening around me. I also appreciate having my own space and working at my own pace. When it comes to my values and the people I care about, I'm incredibly loyal and committed. I'm not a big fan of disagreements or conflicts, and I never try to impose my opinions or values on others.

Introverted, Intuitive, Feeling, and Perceiving (INFP)

I'm idealistic and loyal to my values and the people who matter to me. I strive to live a life that aligns with my values. I'm curious and have a knack for spotting possibilities, often serving as a catalyst for turning ideas into reality. I genuinely seek to understand others and support them in reaching their full potential. I'm adaptable, flexible, and open-minded, unless one of my core values is at stake.

Introverted, Intuitive, Thinking, and Perceiving (INTP)

I'm driven to uncover logical explanations for everything that captures my curiosity. I find myself drawn more to ideas than to social interactions. I often come across as quiet, composed, and open to change, with a remarkable ability to concentrate deeply on solving problems within my field of interest. While I may exhibit skepticism and occasional criticism, my approach is always deeply analytical.

Extraverted, Sensing, Thinking, and Perceiving (ESTP)

I'm someone who's flexible and tolerant, and I like to take a practical approach to get things done. Theoretical and conceptual explanations bore me—I'd rather jump right into action to solve problems. I'm all about living in the present moment, being spontaneous, and enjoying every opportunity to be active with others. I appreciate material comforts and have a sense of style. And you know what? I learn best by doing.

Extraverted, Sensing, Feeling, and Perceiving (ESFP)

I'm outgoing, friendly, and accepting. I absolutely love life, people, and all the little comforts it brings. I thrive on collaborating with others to make things happen. I'm all about bringing common sense and a realistic approach to my work while still managing to make it fun. I'm flexible and spontaneous, always ready to adapt to new people and environments. And you know what? I learn best by diving into new skills alongside others. Let's make things happen together!

Extraverted, Intuitive, Feeling, and Perceiving (ENFP)

I approach life with warmth, enthusiasm, and a vivid imagination, always embracing the endless possibilities it offers. I possess a natural talent for swiftly connecting events and information, confidently navigating based on the patterns I discern. I find great joy in receiving affirmation from others and readily offer appreciation and support in return. My spontaneity, flexibility, and adeptness at improvisation and verbal fluency are integral parts of who I am.

Extraverted, Intuitive, Thinking, and Perceiving (ENTP)

I'm quick, inventive, inspiring, attentive, and candid. I'm resourceful when it comes to solving new and challenging problems. I excel at generating conceptual possibilities and then analyzing them strategically. I'm also adept at understanding other people. Routine bores me, so I rarely do things the same way. I'm always inclined to pursue one new interest after another.

Extraverted, Sensing, Thinking, and Judging (ESTJ)

I'd describe myself as practical, realistic, and matter-of-fact. I'm decisive and like to quickly put my decisions into action. I'm great at organizing projects and people to ensure things get done efficiently. I pay attention to routine details and have a clear set of logical standards that I follow systematically. I'm also quite forceful when it comes to implementing my plans. How can I assist you today?

Extraverted, Sensing, Feeling, and Judging (ESFJ)

I'm a warmhearted, conscientious, and cooperative individual who values harmony in my environment. I work with determination to establish that harmony and enjoy collaborating with others to ensure tasks are completed accurately and on time. I'm loyal and committed, even in small matters. I have a keen eye for noticing what others need in their day-to-day lives and strive to provide it. Most importantly, I want to be appreciated for who I am and the valuable contributions I make.

Extraverted, Intuitive, Feeling, and Judging (ENFJ)

I'm warm, empathetic, responsive, and responsible. I'm really good at understanding how others feel and what they need. I see potential in everyone, and I genuinely want to help them reach their full potential. I can be a catalyst for personal and group growth. I'm loyal, and I appreciate both praise and constructive criticism. I'm also sociable; I enjoy bringing people together; and I can provide inspiring leadership.

Extraverted, Intuitive, Thinking, and Judging (ENTJ)

I'm someone who's frank, decisive, and readily takes on leadership roles. I have a knack for quickly identifying illogical and inefficient procedures and policies, and I enjoy developing and implementing comprehensive systems to solve organizational problems. Long-term planning and goal setting are activities that I find enjoyable, and I'm usually well-informed and well-read. I take pleasure in expanding my knowledge and sharing it with others. When it comes to presenting my ideas, I can be quite forceful.

After reading these descriptions, why not guess at the personality type of your adult child? What category do you feel they fall into?

How Does This Affect How You Interact With Your Adult Child?

Now, let's move deeper into how this understanding can positively impact your interactions and relationship with your adult offspring.

- **Efficient communication:** Knowing your adult child's MBTI type can be a game-changer in communication. For instance, if your child is an Introvert (I), they might appreciate more one-on-one conversations than large gatherings. If they are a Feeler (F), they may prioritize emotional connection in conversations.

Adapting your communication style to suit their preferences can foster a more open and receptive dialogue.

- **Resolution of conflicts:** Conflicts are a natural part of any relationship, but understanding your child's personality type can help you navigate them more effectively. If your child leans toward Thinking (T), they might respond better to logical reasoning and practical solutions. In contrast, a Feeler (F) might require a more empathetic approach, with a focus on understanding and acknowledging their emotions.

- **Setting limits:** Boundaries are crucial in any relationship, and they can vary depending on personality types. If your child is a Perceiver (P), they might appreciate a more flexible approach to boundaries, allowing for spontaneity. Meanwhile, a Judger (J) may prefer well-defined and structured boundaries. By aligning your boundaries with their preferences, you can create a healthier and more harmonious dynamic.

- **Respecting their preferences:** MBTI types can shed light on your child's preferences, values, and priorities. For example, an Introverted (I) child may need solitude to recharge, while an Extraverted (E) child may thrive on social interactions. By respecting these differences, you show that you value and accept them for who they are, which strengthens your relationship.

- **Supporting their growth:** Understanding your child's MBTI type can also guide you in supporting their personal growth and development. For instance, if your child is an Intuitive (N), they may have a thirst for knowledge and exploration. Encourage their curiosity and support opportunities for growth in line with their interests.

- **Establishing a foundation of trust:** Trust is the foundation of any healthy relationship. When you take the time to understand your child's personality type, it demonstrates your commitment to their well-being. This builds trust and reinforces the idea that you're there to support them.

I wanted to offer an example of how our personality types affect how we interact as adults with our children. Let's consider an example with two different MBTI personality types: INTJ (Thinker) and ENFJ (Feeler) in the context of conflict management between a parent and their adult child.

- **Parent (INTJ - Thinker):** The INTJ parent is logical, analytical, and values problem-solving. They approach conflict by seeking facts and practical solutions. In this situation, the INTJ parent may want to sit down with their adult child to discuss the root causes of the conflict, analyze each person's perspective, and propose a clear plan for resolution. They may prioritize finding a rational solution and may struggle to express their emotions.

- **Adult Child (ENFJ - Feeler):** The ENFJ adult child is empathetic, compassionate, and values harmony in relationships. They approach conflict by focusing on emotions and the well-being of all involved. In this case, the ENFJ adult child may desire open communication with their parent, sharing their feelings and seeking emotional validation. They may prioritize understanding each other's emotions and may struggle with the INTJ parent's more analytical approach.

- **Dispute resolution:** The INTJ parent may need to recognize and acknowledge the emotional aspect of the conflict, validating their adult child's feelings. The ENFJ adult child, on the other hand, may benefit from considering practical solutions and being open to the INTJ parent's logical perspective. By finding a balance between emotions and practicality, both parties can work toward a resolution that addresses both the practical issues and emotional needs within their relationship.

I want to remind you that building a healthy relationship with your adult child is a two-way street. It doesn't fall solely on their shoulders. You both must work on it. For this reason, it is a good idea that you also take the MBTI test so both you and your child can understand your personality type as well.

You can find a free resource by visiting: www.16personalities.com

In this chapter, we've explored the remarkable potential that understanding MBTI personality types holds for enhancing our relationships with our adult children. It's a tool that allows us to communicate more effectively, resolve conflicts with empathy, set healthy boundaries, and support our children's growth.

As we journey through the intricate terrain of parenthood, it's important to recognize that the beauty of these personality differences lies in the connections they help us forge. And now, as we eagerly step into the next chapter, we'll explore another fascinating aspect of understanding and nurturing our relationships: love languages.

Discovering how we and our adult children express and receive love can be transformative. It's a key that unlocks the door to more meaningful and harmonious communication.

Chapter 2:

What Is Your Love Language?

As a mother of two grown-up kids myself, I've come to realize that parenting is an ever-evolving journey. The relationships we share with our adult children are unique and constantly changing, and we must adapt and grow alongside them.

In this chapter, we're going to look deep into a fundamental aspect of nurturing these evolving relationships: understanding the concept of love languages. Just like how we used to learn about their favorite toys, games, and foods when they were young, it's equally important to discover how they give and receive love as adults.

You see, as adults, our children develop their own love languages—ways they express and interpret affection. It's not about the language they speak or the words they use, but rather the emotional channels through which they connect with us. Just as we each have our own unique love language, our adult children do too. Recognizing and embracing these love languages can be a powerful tool for strengthening and deepening your bond.

In the following pages, we will explore each of the love languages, how they might manifest in your adult children's lives, and how you can adapt your communication and expressions of love to resonate with their unique preferences.

But before we dive into the specifics, let me share a real-life example to illustrate the importance of understanding love languages.

Meet Sarah and Jack, a mother and son who found themselves at odds despite their deep love for each other. Sarah had always been a nurturing and caring mother, expressing her love through acts of service. She would cook Jack's favorite meals, do his laundry, and run errands for him whenever he needed assistance. However, Jack's primary love language was words of affirmation. He longed to hear his mother say, "I'm proud of you" or "I love you," but Sarah's love was expressed in deeds rather than words. This mismatch caused tension between them, leaving Jack feeling unappreciated and Sarah frustrated.

Through exploring love languages, Sarah and Jack learned to communicate more effectively. Sarah began to express her love verbally, and Jack, in turn, appreciated her acts of service even more. Their relationship blossomed as they bridged this gap in understanding.

By the end of this chapter, you'll be better equipped to speak and understand the unique love languages of your adult children, strengthening the bonds of love that continue to grow between you.

Understanding Love Languages

The concept of love languages was popularized by Dr. Gary Chapman in his book *The 5 Love Languages*. According to his theory, there are five primary love languages that people often adopt for showing and receiving love (Chapman, 2010):

1. Words of affirmation
2. Acts of service
3. Receiving gifts
4. Quality time
5. Physical touch

One of the greatest joys of parenting is the profound love we share with our children. It's a love that evolves and transforms as our kids grow into adults, yet its essence remains unchanged. As our children become independent and navigate their own lives, understanding their love languages can be a powerful tool in maintaining and strengthening our bond with them.

Words of Affirmation

For some of our adult children, words of affirmation are their primary love language. They thrive on verbal expressions of love, praise, and appreciation. A heartfelt "I love you" or "I'm proud of you" can mean the world to them.

- **How it might manifest:** Your child might seek out your encouragement and validation in their career, relationships, or personal achievements. They might appreciate written notes, heartfelt texts, or simply hearing kind words from you regularly.

- **Adapting your communication:** Make it a point to express your love and support through verbal affirmations. Compliment their accomplishments and let them know how much you appreciate their qualities. Keep in mind that the words you use carry weight, so be sincere and specific in your praise.

Acts of Service

Other adult children may value acts of service as their primary love language. They feel loved when someone helps them out or goes the extra mile to make their lives easier.

- **How it might manifest:** Your child may appreciate it when you help with tasks like fixing things around the house, babysitting their kids, or assisting them with errands. They see these actions as tangible expressions of your love.

- **Adapting your communication:** Show your love by offering your assistance and support when they need it. Be proactive in helping them with practical tasks, but always respect their boundaries and independence.

Receiving Gifts

For some individuals, receiving gifts serves as their primary love language. These adult children experience feelings of love when they are given thoughtful, meaningful presents that demonstrate genuine consideration and care.

- **How it might manifest:** Your child might cherish the gifts you give them on special occasions or even appreciate surprise tokens of your love. These gifts may not necessarily be expensive, but they should reflect their interests and preferences.

- **Adapting your communication:** Pay attention to their likes and dislikes, and make an effort to give gifts that hold sentimental value. These gifts don't have to be extravagant; it's the thought and effort that count.

Quality Time

Quality time is another love language that resonates with some adult children. They feel most loved when they have your undivided attention, engaging in meaningful conversations and shared activities.

- **How it might manifest:** Your child may value spending one-on-one time with you, whether it's having a heart-to-heart talk, going for a walk, or simply enjoying a meal together.

- **Adapting your communication:** Be present in the moment when you're with them. Put away distractions, listen actively, and engage in activities they enjoy. Quality time shows them that you prioritize their company.

Physical Touch

Lastly, physical touch is a love language that involves physical closeness and affection. Some adult children feel most loved through hugs, cuddles, or other physical gestures.

- **How it might manifest:** Your child may greet you with a warm hug or enjoy holding hands during a conversation. Physical touch can also be as simple as a pat on the back or a reassuring touch on the arm.

- **Adapting your communication:** Be mindful of their comfort level with physical touch and respect their boundaries. Ensure that your affection is always appropriate and consensual.

Understanding your adult child's love language can help bridge any communication gaps and nurture a deeper connection. Keep in mind that their love language may evolve over time, so staying attuned to their needs and preferences is crucial. Up to this point, we have discussed our adult children's receiving love language. We need to be mindful of how they show love, as it can be a completely different love language.

Let's engage in the story of Mark and his daughter Sarah.

Mark had always been a hardworking and responsible father. His daughter, Sarah, had recently moved out to start her own life as a young adult. They had always shared a close bond, but as Sarah established her independence, Mark noticed that their once-strong connection seemed to be fading.

Sarah was a busy young professional, often working long hours and trying to balance her social life. Whenever they spoke on the phone or visited, their conversations felt shallow, and Mark struggled to understand why their relationship had changed.

One day, Sarah shared with a close friend how she felt distant from her father, despite loving him deeply. Her friend, who had read about love languages, suggested that Sarah talk to her father about it. Intrigued,

Sarah decided to do some research on love languages and see if it could help her reconnect with her dad.

After discovering the concept, Sarah realized that her primary love language was quality time. She cherished meaningful conversations, shared activities, and spending undistracted time with her loved ones. She had grown distant from her father because their interactions had become brief and focused on surface-level topics.

Armed with this newfound understanding, Sarah decided to have an honest conversation with her father. During their next visit, she gently explained her love language and how important quality time was to her. She reassured him that she cherished their relationship but felt they had drifted apart.

Mark, eager to reconnect with his daughter, took her words to heart. He began making an effort to plan special outings, such as hiking trips, museum visits, and even cooking classes, which allowed them to spend quality time together. He also put away his phone during their visits, ensuring he was fully present during their conversations.

As time went on, Mark and Sarah's relationship transformed. They started sharing deeper thoughts, dreams, and emotions with each other. Their bond grew stronger as they rediscovered the joy of quality time spent together.

Sarah felt loved and valued, knowing that her father was making a genuine effort to connect with her in a way that resonated with her love language. Mark, in turn, was grateful for the opportunity to rebuild their relationship and learn more about his adult daughter.

Their story demonstrates how understanding and adapting to your adult child's love language can breathe new life into your relationship. By making the effort to communicate and connect in a way that speaks to their unique preferences, parents can create a deeper and more fulfilling bond with their grown-up children, even as they navigate the challenges of adulthood.

In concluding this chapter, we've explored the transformative power of recognizing and speaking your child's unique love language. As parents, our love for our children is unwavering, but the ways we express that love may differ from one individual to another.

We've learned about the five primary love languages: words of affirmation, acts of service, receiving gifts, quality time, and physical touch, and how they can manifest in your adult child's life. By taking the time to discern their love language, you unlock a deeper level of connection and intimacy in your relationship.

But it doesn't end here. Just as you seek to understand your adult child, they may also want to understand you better. We encourage you to take the free quiz at 5lovelanguages.com/quizzes/love-language to discover your own love language. Understanding how you show and receive love can provide valuable insights into your dynamics as a family.

In the next chapter, we'll delve into a fascinating topic—14 coping styles that we all use in various situations and phases of our lives. These coping styles can significantly impact our relationships with our adult children and ourselves. We'll explore how recognizing and adapting our coping styles can lead to healthier communication, conflict resolution, and a more fulfilling connection with our loved ones.

Chapter 3:
The World of Coping Strategies

In this chapter, we're going to delve into the importance of understanding the coping strategies employed by our adult children. Trust me, this knowledge can be revolutionary in fostering healthier, more meaningful relationships with them.

Coping strategies can be categorized into two main types: adaptive and maladaptive. In adaptive coping, individuals acknowledge the source of their stress and take proactive measures to either modify the situation itself or alter their responses to it. On the other hand, maladaptive coping occurs when individuals avoid addressing the underlying problem or stressor altogether. This chapter will focus on adaptive coping strategies.

As you read through this chapter, consider taking the Brief Coping Orientation to Problems Experienced Inventory (COPE) questionnaire and encourage your adult children to do the same. This self-awareness can be a catalyst for more empathetic and supportive relationships as we adapt to the changing dynamics of our parent–adult child connections.

www.psychologytoday.com/sg/tests/career/coping-stress-management-skills-test.com

Why we should understand coping strategies:

- **Empathy and connection:** Understanding our adult children's coping strategies allows us to connect with them on a deeper level. When we comprehend how they deal with life's challenges, it fosters empathy. We can put ourselves in their shoes and genuinely understand what they're going through.

- **Productive communication:** This is the cornerstone of any healthy relationship. When we know how our adult children cope with stress, anxiety, or conflicts, we can tailor our communication style to suit their needs. This ensures that our conversations are more productive and less stressful for both parties.

- **Reducing misunderstandings:** Misunderstandings often arise when we assume that everyone copes with stress or conflict the same way we do. By understanding our children's coping strategies, we can avoid jumping to conclusions or misinterpreting their actions and reactions.

- **Building trust:** Trust is the foundation of any strong relationship. When we show an interest in understanding our adult children's coping mechanisms, it sends a powerful message that we care about their well-being and respect their individuality. This builds trust and reinforces the parent–child bond.

This knowledge can improve your relationship:

- **Validation and assistance:** When we acknowledge and respect our adult children's coping strategies, we validate their feelings and choices. This support can empower them to cope more effectively, knowing that we stand by their side.

- **Problem resolution:** Understanding how our children cope can be helpful in conflict resolution. For example, if your child tends to use humor to cope, you can approach conflicts with a lighter tone, making it easier for them to engage in conversations.

- **Setting healthy limits:** Effective boundary-setting is vital in any relationship. By understanding your adult child's coping mechanisms, you can establish boundaries that respect their needs and help maintain a healthy balance between independence and support.

- **Adapting to their needs:** Our children's needs evolve as they grow and face different life challenges. Understanding their coping strategies enables us to adapt our parenting approach as they transition into adulthood.

- **Supporting their growth:** Ultimately, our goal as parents is to help our children grow into confident and resilient adults. By understanding their coping styles, we can provide guidance and support that aligns with their unique needs, facilitating personal growth and self-awareness.

Before we jump into the specifics, remember this: Our children's coping styles are not a reflection of our parenting. Each individual develops their own unique ways to navigate life's challenges, and these strategies are often rooted in their own experiences, personalities, and the ever-changing world around them.

Problem-Focused Coping

Problem-focused coping involves taking actions to address or eliminate the root causes of stress. This approach is effective when there is some level of control over the stress-inducing situation. Let's explore how problem-focused coping strategies can be applied to real-life scenarios within the context of parent–adult child relationships:

Scenario 1: Frequent Conflicts Between an Adult Child and Parent

Possible problem-focused responses:

- Initiate open communication with your adult child to understand their perspective.
- Look into family therapy or counseling to work through underlying issues and improve the relationship.
- Set clear, healthy boundaries and expectations to reduce conflicts.
- If necessary, consider temporarily reducing contact to create space for both parties to reflect and reset.

Scenario 2: Parenting an Adult Child With Financial Struggles

Possible problem-focused responses:

- Help your adult child make a budget and plan for their money.
- Advise them to look for a job or ways to move up in their career.
- Give advice on handling debts and learning more about money.
- Check out ways they can learn more or get more skills for better jobs.

Emotion-Focused Coping

Stress is an inevitable part of life, and sometimes we find ourselves in situations where we have little control over the underlying stressors. In such cases, emotion-focused coping strategies become valuable tools to.help us manage our emotional responses. These strategies don't necessarily change the situation, but they can alter the way we react to it.

Now, let's explore some examples of emotion-focused coping strategies within the context of parent–adult child relationships:

Scenario 1: Coping With a Parent's Serious Illness

Possible emotion-focused responses:

- Find trustworthy medical information to learn more about the illness.
- Join a group or online community to talk about your experiences and feelings.

- Write in a journal to let out your feelings and thoughts and help you deal with them.

Scenario 2: Navigating Stressful Family Gatherings

Possible emotion-focused responses:

- Use calming methods like deep breathing or mindfulness to handle social anxiety.
- Go to the event with a close friend or family member to get emotional support.
- Think of things to talk about or ways to start conversations to make social interactions easier and reduce anxiety.

In these examples, emotion-focused coping strategies aim to help both the adult child and the parent manage their emotional responses to challenging situations. While these strategies may not alter the external circumstances causing stress, they can provide valuable tools for regulating emotions and enhancing overall well-being.

Adaptive Coping Strategies

Now, as we move deeper into adaptive coping strategies, we will focus on those that are looked at as "healthy" or adaptive coping strategies. We will break these down into specific coping strategies.

Active Coping (Problem-Focused)

Active coping involves taking direct and assertive actions to address stressors or challenges actively. It focuses on problem-solving, seeking solutions, and actively managing stressful situations rather than passively reacting to them.

Impact on behavior and interactions:

- **Proactive approach:** Adult children who adopt an active coping style tend to take a proactive and assertive approach when facing challenges. They don't wait for problems to resolve themselves but take action to address them.
- **Problem-solving orientation:** This coping style emphasizes problem-solving skills. Adult children actively seek solutions, analyze options, and make strategic decisions to resolve difficulties.
- **Effective stress management:** Active coping is associated with effective stress management. It allows adult children to regain a sense of control over their lives and reduce the impact of stressors.

Impact on relationship and communication:

- **Productive communication:** Active coping promotes effective communication within the parent–child relationship. Adult children are likely to engage in clear and assertive discussions when addressing challenges or concerns.
- **Collaborative approach:** This coping style often encourages a collaborative approach to problem-solving. Parents and adult children may work together to find solutions and make decisions.
- **Conflict management:** This is typically more efficient when individuals use active coping. It encourages open dialogue, assertiveness, and a focus on finding mutually agreeable solutions.
- **Mutual respect:** Active coping fosters mutual respect within the relationship. Parents may appreciate their adult child's ability to take charge and make informed decisions.
- **Potential misunderstanding:** When your adult child leans into this type of coping strategy, there is the potential for misunderstanding. You may feel your child seems to lack

emotion or appears to be heartless because they are so focused on solving the problem at hand.

Use of Informational Support (Problem-Focused)

The use of informational support coping style involves seeking knowledge, advice, or information from various sources, including experts, resources, or trusted individuals, to better understand and address a particular challenge or stressor. It emphasizes the importance of informed decision-making.

Impact on behavior and interactions:

- **Research-oriented:** Adult children who adopt the use of informational support tend to be research-oriented and proactive in seeking information. They may invest time in gathering facts and data relevant to their challenges.

- **Informed decision-making:** This coping style prioritizes informed decision-making. Adult children are likely to make choices based on the insights and knowledge they have acquired through research.

- **Resourcefulness:** Individuals who practice the use of informational support often display resourcefulness. They are skilled at identifying valuable resources and experts who can provide guidance.

Impact on relationship and communication:

- **Clear communication:** The use of informational support encourages effective communication. Adult children may engage in clear and informative discussions with their parents, sharing the information they have gathered.

- **Mutual learning:** It can foster mutual learning within the parent–child relationship. Parents may also benefit from the information and insights their adult child acquires.

- **Problem-solving orientation:** This coping style promotes a problem-solving orientation in relationships. Adult children may seek practical solutions to challenges and communicate them effectively.

- **Enhanced trust:** Seeking informational support can enhance trust within the parent–child relationship. When parents see their child taking initiative and making informed decisions, it can strengthen trust and confidence.

- **Potential misunderstanding:** This may arise if your child adapts this coping strategy and takes significant time when making decisions. You may feel that they aren't making decisions fast enough for your liking, that they don't take enough risks, or that they are not spontaneous.

Positive Reframing (Problem-Focused)

Positive reframing involves consciously changing one's perspective to find positive aspects or opportunities within challenging situations. It entails looking beyond the initial negative or stressful aspects and focusing on the potential for growth, learning, or positive outcomes.

Impact on behavior and interactions:

- **Optimistic outlook:** Adult children who adopt a positive reframing coping style tend to maintain an optimistic outlook even when faced with difficulties. They actively seek the silver lining in challenging situations.

- **Resilience:** Positive reframing can enhance resilience. It helps individuals bounce back from adversity more effectively by emphasizing the potential for personal growth and strength.

- **Solution-focused:** Those who practice positive reframing are often solution-focused. They look for constructive ways to address challenges and are open to exploring different approaches.

Impact on relationship and communication:

- **Positive atmosphere:** The positive reframing coping style can create a positive and uplifting atmosphere in interactions with parents. It fosters optimism and a sense of hope.

- **Shared positivity**: Sharing positive reframing with parents can lead to shared positivity within the parent–child relationship. It can serve as a source of mutual support and inspiration.

- **Productive communication:** Positive reframing encourages constructive and effective communication. Adult children may approach difficult conversations with a focus on finding solutions and highlighting opportunities for growth.

- **Dispute resolution:** This may be more productive and less emotionally charged in relationships where positive reframing is employed. It promotes a problem-solving mindset.

- **Potential misunderstanding:** As a parent of an adult child who adopts this coping style, it can lead to misunderstandings if your child seems optimistic at all times. This can feel unrealistic, or even frustrating and off-putting for some.

By supporting and embracing your adult child's positive reframing coping style, you can contribute to a more optimistic, constructive, and mutually supportive parent–child relationship. Encourage open communication, shared positivity, and a focus on solutions to strengthen your bond.

Planning (Problem-Focused)

The planning coping style involves taking a proactive and structured approach to managing stress and challenges. It entails setting clear goals, making organized plans, and utilizing problem-solving strategies to address difficulties effectively.

Impact on behavior and interactions:

- **Goal-oriented:** Adult children who adopt a planning coping style tend to be goal-oriented and organized in their actions. They identify specific objectives and create step-by-step plans to achieve them.

- **Problem-solving:** This coping style emphasizes problem-solving skills. Adult children use analytical thinking and logical strategies to address challenges and find solutions.

- **Active approach:** Planning involves taking an active and hands-on approach to managing stress. Adult children actively seek ways to mitigate difficulties and minimize their impact.

Impact on relationship and communication:

- **Efficient communication:** Adult children who use a planning coping style may excel in clear and effective communication. They are skilled at expressing their needs, concerns, and solutions.

- **Collaborative approach:** Planning often promotes a collaborative approach to problem-solving. In interactions with their parents, adult children may seek input and collaboration to address family issues.

- **Mutual respect:** The planning coping style encourages mutual respect in relationships. Parents and adult children may appreciate each other's ability to approach challenges with logic and problem-solving skills.

- **Dispute management:** This may be more structured and less emotionally charged in relationships with individuals who adopt the planning coping style. It often leads to more efficient resolutions.

- **Potential misunderstanding:** If your adult child uses this coping strategy, you may find yourself frustrated by their constant need to plan. It can be time-consuming, and if you are spontaneous, this can lead to misunderstandings.

By supporting and collaborating with your adult child's planning coping style, you can contribute to a more constructive and effective parent–child relationship. Emphasize clear communication, mutual respect, and shared problem-solving efforts to strengthen your bond.

Emotional Support (Emotion-Focused)

The emotional support coping style involves seeking and relying on emotional support from others, such as friends, family, or a support network, to manage stress, cope with challenges, and process emotions. It entails sharing feelings, seeking comfort, and connecting with supportive individuals.

Impact on behavior and interactions:

- **Seeking comfort:** Adult children who adopt an emotional support coping style are likely to reach out to others when facing difficulties. They seek comfort, empathy, and understanding from those they trust.

- **Expressive communication:** This coping style encourages expressive communication. Adult children may openly share their thoughts and feelings, allowing them to process emotions and find solace in sharing their experiences.

- **Building strong connections:** Seeking emotional support fosters strong connections with individuals who provide that support. This can lead to deeper and more meaningful relationships within their social network.

Impact on relationship and communication:

- **Positive interactions:** Emotional support coping can contribute to positive and empathetic interactions between parents and adult children. Both parties may feel comfortable discussing emotions and offering support.

- **Shared experiences:** Sharing emotional experiences can deepen the bond between parents and adult children. It fosters a sense of understanding and mutual care.

- **Communication of needs:** Adult children who adopt this coping style may effectively communicate their emotional needs to their parents. They express when they require support and may also offer support in return.

- **Dispute resolution:** Emotional support coping can contribute to healthier dispute resolution. It promotes open dialogue and empathetic listening, which can lead to better problem-solving strategies.

Overall, understanding and respecting your adult child's emotional support coping style can contribute to a more empathetic and supportive parent–child relationship. Encourage open communication, express your love and support, and be receptive to their emotional needs to strengthen your bond.

Venting (Emotion-Focused)

Venting as a coping style involves expressing and releasing pent-up emotions, frustrations, or stress through verbal or written communication. It often entails sharing feelings, grievances, or concerns with the goal of finding relief or emotional release.

Impact on behavior and interactions:

- **Emotional release:** Adult children who adopt a venting coping style may engage in emotional release by openly expressing their feelings and thoughts. Venting provides an outlet for them to unburden themselves.

- **Catharsis:** Venting can serve as a form of catharsis, allowing individuals to purge negative emotions and reduce stress levels. It may help them feel lighter and more emotionally balanced.

- **Processing emotions:** Venting can facilitate the process of processing and understanding one's emotions. It can help individuals gain clarity about their feelings and experiences.

Impact on relationship and communication:

- **Open communication:** A venting coping style can create a safe space for adult children and their parents to openly share their thoughts and emotions, fostering open and honest communication.
- **Shared bond:** Sharing emotional experiences and concerns can strengthen the connection between parents and adult children, fostering a profound sense of mutual support and understanding.
- **Conflict resolution:** Venting can be a part of conflict resolution. It allows adult children to express their concerns and grievances, potentially leading to productive discussions and resolutions.
- **Potential for misunderstanding:** Venting may sometimes involve expressing strong emotions, which can be intense for both parties.

In summary, supporting your adult child's venting coping style can contribute to a more open and understanding parent–child relationship. It allows for the free expression of emotions and can promote emotional bonding and mutual support. However, it's essential to be mindful of boundaries and ensure that venting remains a constructive and healthy way to cope with stress and emotions.

Humor (Emotion-Focused)

The humor coping style involves using humor, laughter, and wit as a way to manage stress, alleviate tension, and cope with challenging situations. It often involves finding amusement or irony in life's difficulties.

Impact on behavior and interactions:

- **Light-hearted approach:** Adult children who employ a humor coping style tend to approach stressful situations with a light-hearted and playful attitude. They may use humor as a means of defusing tension.

- **Stress reduction:** Humor can be an effective stress-reduction tool. It can help reduce the intensity of difficult situations, making them more manageable and less overwhelming.

- **Enhanced resilience:** Those who use humor to cope may demonstrate greater resilience in the face of adversity. They are more likely to bounce back from challenges with a positive outlook.

Impact on relationship and communication:

- **Positive atmosphere:** A humor coping style can create a positive and enjoyable atmosphere in interactions with parents. It can make communication more pleasant and less confrontational.

- **Easier problem solving:** Adult children who use humor may be more skilled at resolving problems through peaceful means. They can use humor to disarm potentially contentious situations and find common ground.

- **Shared laughter:** Shared laughter and humor can be a bonding experience. Engaging in humorous exchanges with your adult child can strengthen the parent–child relationship.

- **Productive communication:** Humor can be an effective tool for conveying thoughts and feelings. Adult children may use humor to express themselves in a nonthreatening manner, making it easier to communicate openly.

- **Potential misunderstanding:** It should come as no surprise that if your child uses humor as a coping strategy, it can lead to misunderstandings. If a serious situation presents itself, you would expect humor to take a backseat. Understanding that this is how they cope can avoid these misunderstandings.

Acceptance (Emotion-Focused)

The acceptance coping style involves acknowledging and coming to terms with difficult or challenging situations without attempting to change or control them actively. It entails embracing the reality of the situation and finding inner peace and contentment within it.

Impact on behavior and interactions:

- **Embracing reality:** Adult children who adopt an acceptance coping style tend to approach stressful situations with a sense of calm and composure. They acknowledge that some aspects of life are beyond their control and focus on adapting to the circumstances.

- **Reduced resistance:** Instead of resisting or fighting against challenging situations, individuals who practice acceptance coping tend to let go of the need for control. This can lead to reduced stress and anxiety, as they are not constantly battling against circumstances.

- **Resilience:** Acceptance can foster resilience, as it allows individuals to bounce back from adversity more effectively. They are less likely to dwell on negative emotions and are more open to finding positive aspects or opportunities for growth within challenges.

Impact on relationship and communication:

- **Clear communication:** Adult children who adopt an acceptance coping style may be more adept at engaging in calm and rational discussions with their parents. They are less likely to become defensive or confrontational in difficult conversations.

- **Empathy and understanding:** Acceptance can lead to greater empathy and understanding of others, including parents. Adult children may be more attuned to their parents' perspectives and emotions, which can enhance their communication.

- **Less stress in interactions:** When an adult child accepts that they cannot control every aspect of their relationship with their parents, interactions tend to be less stressful. Acceptance can reduce the pressure to meet unrealistic expectations or change the parent's behavior.

- **Conflict resolution:** Those who practice acceptance may approach conflicts with a more cooperative and collaborative mindset. They are more likely to seek compromise and mutually beneficial solutions.

- **Potential misunderstanding:** If your adult child uses acceptance as a coping strategy and you have a strong personality, you may find yourself feeling frustrated. Assuming that this means your child is not strong and is simply a pushover can lead to potential misunderstandings.

Overall, understanding and respecting your adult child's acceptance coping style can lead to a more harmonious and less stressful parent–child relationship. By embracing their approach to challenges and maintaining open communication, you can nurture a strong and enduring bond.

Religion (Emotion-Focused)

Religious coping involves turning to one's faith or spirituality as a source of strength, comfort, and guidance in times of stress, difficulty, or crisis. This coping style relies on religious beliefs, practices, and values to navigate life's challenges.

Impact on behavior and interactions:

- **Seeking guidance from faith:** Adult children who adopt a religious coping style may seek guidance and solace through religious texts, prayers, or rituals. They may turn to their faith community for support and guidance.

- **Positive coping mechanism:** For many, religious coping can be a positive and adaptive way to manage stress. It may provide a sense of purpose, hope, and resilience during difficult times.

- **Community engagement:** Engagement with a religious community can lead to increased social connections and support. This can be particularly beneficial when an adult child faces challenges or needs emotional assistance.

Impact on relationship and communication:

- **Shared values:** If both the parent and adult child share the same religious beliefs, it can strengthen the parent–child bond. A shared faith can serve as a foundation for common values, traditions, and rituals.

- **Conflict management:** Religious coping can affect the way conflicts are approached. Some individuals may rely on prayer or spiritual guidance to resolve conflicts, while others may seek advice from religious leaders.

- **Communication style:** Adult children who rely on religious coping may incorporate religious language or references in their conversations with their parents. This can be a form of sharing their beliefs and seeking emotional support.

- **Potential misunderstanding:** This coping style can lead to misunderstandings if you feel that they hide behind their faith, using it as an excuse or a shield.

Overall, understanding and respecting your adult child's religious coping style can foster a more empathetic and supportive parent–child relationship. By acknowledging the significance of faith in their life and being open to conversations about it, you can strengthen your connection and provide valuable emotional support when needed.

In this chapter, we've explored the diverse coping strategies that adult children may employ when facing life's challenges. By delving into these adaptive coping styles, we've gained insights into how our children's behavior, interactions, relationships, and communication can be influenced. Remember that these coping mechanisms reflect their unique ways of managing stress and navigating adulthood.

As parents, understanding these coping styles helps us approach our relationships with empathy, patience, and support. It is important to be mindful that this knowledge is also beneficial to you. By recognizing that our children's choices are often shaped by their coping strategies, we can foster stronger bonds and more open lines of communication. Having this understanding allows us to interact with our adult child in a more positive and effective manner.

In the next chapter, we'll delve into the realm of maladaptive coping strategies—those that may raise concerns and affect our relationships in less constructive ways. By understanding both adaptive and maladaptive coping mechanisms, we'll be better equipped to navigate the complex journey of parenting adult children and fostering healthier relationships.

Chapter 3.1:
Maladaptive Coping Strategies

As we explore the world of parenting adult children, it's important to understand the maladaptive coping strategies they may use. In this chapter, we'll look into these strategies, why our adult children may rely on them, and why it's crucial for us as parents to understand their significance.

It is important to understand that these maladaptive coping strategies are not born out of a desire to thwart our parental guidance or cause us distress. Rather, they emerge as responses to the unique pressures and demands they face in their lives. And as parents, understanding these strategies is not only a testament to our unwavering support, but it's also a vital step toward fostering healthy, open, and meaningful relationships with our adult children.

Maladaptive Coping Strategies

Self-Blame (Emotion-Focused)

Self-blame coping involves an individual directing blame and criticism toward themselves when faced with stress, challenges, or conflicts. Instead of externalizing the problem or situation, they internalize it and believe that they are responsible for the difficulties they encounter.

Impact on behavior and interactions:

- **Excessive self-criticism:** Adult children who employ self-blame coping may be excessively critical of themselves. They may perceive themselves as the root cause of problems, which can lead to feelings of guilt and shame.

- **Avoidance of responsibility:** In an attempt to shoulder the blame, they may encompass responsibility for the actions or decisions, even when the fault lies elsewhere. This acceptance of responsibility belonging elsewhere can hinder personal growth and problem-solving.

Impact on relationship and communication:

- **Difficulty in expressing needs:** Adult children who engage in self-blame may struggle to communicate their needs or concerns to their parents. They might feel unworthy of help or support, believing that they should handle everything on their own.

- **Low self-esteem:** Continuous self-blame can erode self-esteem and self-worth, making them doubt their abilities and value. This may manifest in a lack of confidence in various aspects of life.

- **Tendency to apologize excessively:** They may apologize frequently, even for matters beyond their control or unrelated to them. This can lead to a strained dynamic, as parents may become confused or frustrated by constant apologies.

- **Miscommunication:** The internalized self-blame can lead to misunderstandings and miscommunication. Parents may perceive their adult child's self-criticism as a sign of unresponsiveness or disinterest, while the child may feel misunderstood or judged.

- **Impact on parent–child bond:** Over time, persistent self-blame can strain the parent–child relationship. Parents may worry about their child's well-being and self-esteem, while the child may distance themselves emotionally to avoid burdening their parents with their perceived failures.

By fostering a supportive and understanding environment, parents can help their adult children shift away from self-blame coping toward more adaptive and healthier ways of managing stress and challenges, ultimately strengthening their relationship.

Self-Distraction (Avoidant)

Self-distraction coping involves diverting one's attention away from stressors or challenges by engaging in activities or behaviors that provide temporary relief or an escape from the source of stress. It often entails seeking solace in distractions to temporarily alleviate emotional distress.

Impact on behavior and interactions:

- **Temporary relief:** Adult children who adopt a self-distraction coping style may temporarily find relief from stress or emotional distress through engaging in various distractions or activities.

- **Escape mechanism:** Self-distraction can serve as an escape mechanism, allowing individuals to momentarily step away from the intensity of their stressors or emotions.

- **Avoidance of confrontation:** In some cases, self-distraction may be used to avoid confronting or addressing the root causes of stress or difficulties, as it offers a temporary reprieve.

Impact on relationship and communication:

- **Limited communication:** When adult children rely heavily on self-distraction, it may limit their willingness or ability to communicate openly with their parents about their stressors or concerns.

- **Potential for misunderstanding:** Parents may perceive the use of self-distraction as avoidance or lack of engagement in the relationship. This can lead to potential misunderstandings or strained interactions.

- **Emotional distance:** Overreliance on self-distraction can create emotional distance between parents and adult children. The avoidance of discussing stressors may hinder emotional intimacy.

- **Communication challenges:** If self-distraction becomes the primary coping mechanism, it may hinder effective communication regarding family issues or challenges that require discussion and resolution.

Overall, supporting your adult child's self-distraction coping style involves striking a balance between respecting their need for temporary relief and fostering open communication. Encourage them to find healthy coping strategies that balance self-distraction with addressing underlying stressors when necessary to maintain a strong and connected parent–child relationship.

Denial (Avoidant)

The denial coping style involves consciously or unconsciously refusing to acknowledge or accept the presence of stressors, difficulties, or emotions. It often entails avoiding or minimizing the significance of challenging situations as a means of reducing emotional distress.

Impact on behavior and interactions:

- **Avoidance of reality:** Adult children who adopt a denial coping style may actively avoid or deny the reality of their stressors or emotions. They may convince themselves that the problems or feelings do not exist.

- **Temporary relief:** Denial can provide temporary relief from emotional distress, as it allows individuals to distance themselves from the intensity of their stressors or challenges.

- **Avoidance of confrontation:** This coping style may be used to avoid confronting or addressing the root causes of stress or difficulties. It offers a temporary escape from uncomfortable or distressing truths.

Impact on relationship and communication:

- **Limited communication:** An adult child relying heavily on denial may be less willing to communicate openly with their parents about their stressors or concerns. They may downplay or avoid discussing issues altogether.

- **Potential for misunderstanding:** Parents may perceive the use of denial as a lack of engagement or avoidance of the relationship's challenges. This can lead to misunderstandings or strained interactions.

- **Emotional distance:** Overreliance on denial can create emotional distance between parents and adult children. Avoiding discussions about stressors may hinder emotional intimacy.

- **Communication barriers:** If denial becomes the primary coping mechanism, it can create significant communication barriers when it comes to addressing family issues or challenges that require discussion and resolution.

It's important to strike a balance between respecting their need for temporary denial and fostering open communication when they are ready to address underlying stressors. Encourage them to find healthier ways to cope that allow them to acknowledge and manage their challenges when necessary to maintain a strong and connected parent–child relationship.

Substance Use (Avoidant)

The substance use coping style involves turning to substances such as alcohol, drugs, or other addictive behaviors as a means of coping with stress, emotional distress, or challenging situations. It often entails using substances to numb or escape negative emotions temporarily.

Impact on behavior and interactions:

- **Dependency:** Adult children who adopt a substance use coping style may become dependent on substances to manage stress. They may use substances regularly to cope with emotional pain or discomfort.

- **Escapism:** Substance use serves as a form of escapism, allowing individuals to temporarily escape from the intensity of their stressors, difficulties, or emotions.
- **Risk of addiction:** This coping style carries a significant risk of addiction and substance abuse issues, as it can lead to a cycle of increased reliance on substances to cope.

Impact on relationship and communication:

- **Communication breakdown:** Substance use can lead to communication breakdown within the parent–child relationship. Adult children may become less open or communicative as they prioritize substance use over discussions.
- **Strained interactions:** The use of substances may lead to strained interactions with parents, as it can affect mood, behavior, and judgment. Parents may feel concerned or distant from their adult child.
- **Risk of conflict:** Substance use can be a source of conflict between parents and adult children, particularly if it leads to negative consequences or family tension.
- **Lack of emotional connection:** Overreliance on substance use may hinder emotional connection and intimacy within the relationship, as emotions may be masked or numbed by substances.

It's crucial to approach the issue of substance use with compassion, empathy, and a focus on helping your adult child seek healthier coping strategies. While it may be challenging, maintaining a supportive and nonjudgmental stance can contribute to the possibility of recovery and a stronger parent–child relationship.

Behavioral Disengagement (Avoidant)

Behavioral disengagement coping involves withdrawing or disengaging from stressors, challenges, or difficult emotions by physically or mentally distancing oneself from the situation. It often entails avoiding or ignoring stressors rather than actively addressing them.

Impact on behavior and interactions:

- **Withdrawal:** Adult children who adopt a behavioral disengagement coping style may withdraw from the situation or become emotionally distant. They may isolate themselves or avoid activities that trigger stress.

- **Inactivity:** Behavioral disengagement often leads to inactivity or a lack of motivation to address stressors actively. Adult children may become passive in their approach to difficulties.

- **Avoidance:** This coping style involves the avoidance of confronting or dealing with stressors directly. Adult children may prefer to bury their feelings or distract themselves from the source of stress.

Impact on relationship and communication:

- **Limited interaction:** Behavioral disengagement can result in limited interaction between parents and adult children. The adult child may become less communicative or less willing to engage in family activities.

- **Emotional distance:** Overreliance on this coping style can create emotional distance within the parent–child relationship. The avoidance of discussing stressors may hinder emotional intimacy.

- **Lack of conflict resolution:** Behavioral disengagement can impede conflict resolution within the relationship, as the adult child may avoid addressing issues or expressing their concerns.

- **Communication barriers:** If behavioral disengagement becomes the primary coping mechanism, it can create significant communication barriers when it comes to addressing family issues or challenges that require discussion and resolution.

Balancing support with respect for their boundaries and coping style is essential in helping your adult child gradually transition to more constructive coping strategies. The key is to maintain a patient and nonjudgmental approach, fostering a space where they feel safe to open up and engage in healthy communication and problem-solving.

As we conclude this chapter about maladaptive coping strategies, it's important to reflect on the valuable lessons we have learned. We have examined the complex ways in which our adult children deal with life's challenges, and we now understand that their coping mechanisms go beyond superficial behaviors. Instead, they are intricate responses to the world they live in.

Understanding these coping strategies does not mean we are approving or encouraging destructive behaviors. Instead, it is a way to develop compassion and empathy. Our adult children are not intentionally confusing us; they are dealing with their own pressures, anxieties, and circumstances. As parents, our role is not to judge but to offer support and guidance.

In the upcoming chapter, we will explore the psychological changes that children experience as they transition from childhood to adulthood. This journey involves significant shifts in their identity, beliefs, and values. By understanding these psychological transformations, we can navigate the complexities of our evolving relationships more effectively.

Let's take the knowledge from this chapter with us, not as a burden but as a tool to build healthier connections with our adult children. By approaching with open hearts and a commitment to understanding, we can navigate the path that helps us comprehend the psychological changes they go through.

Chapter 4:
The Psychological Changes in Adult Children and the Impact on Parental Roles

In this chapter, we are about to embark on an important exploration of the profound psychological changes that our children go through as they transition from their teenage years into adulthood. Additionally, we'll look into the evolving role we, as parents, play in their lives during this transformative period.

I know from personal experience that this transition can be both exhilarating and daunting. It's a time when our children spread their wings and embark on their own unique paths. The once-familiar landscape of their childhood is now transforming into uncharted territory, and as parents, we must adapt and grow alongside them.

Let's begin by acknowledging a fundamental truth: We cannot expect to have the same relationship with our adult children as we did when they were younger. The dynamics are shifting, and it's important that we understand and embrace these changes to foster healthy and meaningful connections.

I want to help unravel the mysteries of our children's changing minds and hearts, all while discovering how our role as parents evolves into that of mentors and consultants.

From Teen to Adult: Navigating the Psychological Changes

As our children step into adulthood, they don't just grow physically. They take a psychological journey as well. These changes can be both exhilarating and confusing, and it's important for us to understand what's happening in their minds:

- **Identity exploration:** During this phase, your child is trying to figure out who they are. They may experiment with various identities, hobbies, and even relationships. This is a time of self-discovery, and sometimes it might seem like they're in constant flux. It is important that we give them space and allow them to figure this one out on their own without criticism or judgment.
    - **Real-life example:** Charles has a son, James, who went through a phase where he explored different hobbies, from playing guitar to painting. It was like he was searching for something that truly resonated with him. Charles did his best to keep his opinions to himself and even offered to take an art class with him.
- **Independence and autonomy:** Your child's desire for independence increases. They want to make their own decisions, manage their finances, and have more control over their lives. This can lead to clashes if not handled with understanding.
    - **Real-life example:** Sarah, a mother of two, shared her experience. Her daughter, Emily, wanted to move out and live on her own after college. Although it was tough for Sarah, she respected Emily's need for independence and supported her in finding her own place.
- **Emotional rollercoaster:** Young adults often grapple with emotional ups and downs. They may be more assertive and yet vulnerable, trying to navigate adult emotions, relationships, and responsibilities.
- **Statistic:** Adults between the ages of 18 and 25 are almost twice as likely as teenagers to experience anxiety and depression, as per the latest data from the Making Caring Common project (**Kindelan, 2023**). We need to be aware that this is a difficult time emotionally and mentally for our children

as they move from a teen to an adult. Being available and supportive is important. Be an example, mirror vulnerability, and don't be afraid to show your child that therapy is empowering. Most times, they just need to know you are there if they need to talk without judgment.

Changing Roles as Parents

As our children undergo these psychological changes, our roles as parents need to adapt:

- **Maintaining a supportive presence:** While they seek independence, our children still need our support. This support can come in various forms, from offering a listening ear to providing a safety net during challenging times.

- **Communication is key:** Effective communication becomes even more crucial during this transition. Encourage open dialogue, active listening, and empathy. Be patient when they share their struggles or successes.

In this evolving relationship, it's essential to understand that we are not losing our children; we are gaining adult friends. While the journey can be rocky at times, it is also filled with opportunities for growth, connection, and shared experiences.

From Parent to Mentor

Our role as a parent evolves as our children grow, and it's important that we adapt with grace, support, and understanding. Let's review some great ways we can make that happen:

- **Treat them as equals:** One of the first steps in transitioning from parent to mentor is to treat your adult children as equals. This doesn't mean abandoning your role as a parent, but recognizing that mutual respect is the foundation of any healthy relationship. By showing them respect, you'll earn it in return.

- **Case study:** Hilary has a son, Mark, with whom she had a heated disagreement about a life choice he was making. Instead of insisting she was right, she listened to his perspective and respected his decision, even though she didn't fully agree. Their relationship became stronger because of it.

- **Learn from them:** As parents, we often believe we have all the answers. But remember, our children can teach us too! They bring fresh perspectives, innovative ideas, and new experiences into our lives. Don't be afraid to learn from them and embrace their wisdom.

  - **Personal story:** Elaine has an adult daughter who introduced her to mindfulness meditation, which has had a profound impact on her well-being. This is not something she would have ever explored on her own. Elaine is grateful for the lessons she's learned from her daughter.

- **Apologize when wrong:** Parents aren't infallible, and it's important to set an example of taking responsibility for our actions. If you make a mistake, apologize sincerely. It shows your adult children that it's okay to admit when they're wrong too.

  - **Expert opinion:** Psychologists recommend acknowledging your mistakes as a way to model accountability for your adult children (**Travers, 2023**).

- **Remember they are adults now:** It's crucial to acknowledge that your children are no longer the little kids you once knew. They have their own lives, dreams, and aspirations. Embrace their adulthood and respect their autonomy.

  - **Real-life example:** Jim is a father whose son moved to a different city for a job. He struggled with this for quite some time, feeling like a piece of him was missing and wanting to tell his son to move back. Although he misses his son terribly, he respects his choice and his need for independence.

- **Change is inevitable:** Change is a constant in life, and our children growing up is one of the most significant changes we'll experience. Embrace change with grace and an open heart, knowing that your child is embarking on their own journey.
  - **Personal experience:** Tamara has twin daughters, and their world was her world. They did everything together, so when the day came for them to move out on their own, her heart ached. She hadn't prepared herself for this next step in the journey. Taking a step back, she remembered when she took that leap at their age. The change in perspective allowed her to start enjoying their excitement for the future. Accepting that her children were no longer dependent on her was a process, but it allowed her to appreciate their newfound independence.

- **Respect goes both ways:** Just as you expect respect from your adult children, remember to treat them with the same respect you'd want. Respect is a two-way street and forms the foundation of a healthy mentorship.
  - **Case study:** Meet Lisa and her son, Jake. As a teenager, Jake was known for his rebellious streak, often clashing with his parents over rules and boundaries. However, as Jake transitioned into adulthood, Lisa realized that she needed to shift her approach. She began treating him with more respect, listening to his opinions, and valuing his perspective. Instead of imposing her views on him, she started engaging in open and respectful conversations. Over time, something remarkable happened. Jake, feeling respected and valued by his mother, reciprocated that respect. He began seeking Lisa's advice and guidance voluntarily. They developed a closer bond built on trust, and Lisa found herself not just as a parent but also as a trusted mentor in Jake's life. It's a testament to the transformative power of

respect in building strong connections with adult children.

- **Be a role model:** Show your adult children what resilience, strength, and perseverance look like. Be an example of the qualities you hope to see in them. Your actions will speak louder than words.
    - **Research-backed information:** Studies have shown that children are more likely to emulate their parents' behavior and values as adults (**Schofield et al., 2012).**
- **Balancing parent and friend:** Finding the balance between being a parent and a friend to your grown-up kids can be challenging. It's okay to be friendly, but remember that you're still their parent. Open communication can help strike this balance.
    - **Community support:** Joining parenting support groups or seeking advice from other parents going through similar transitions can provide valuable insights.
- **The art of letting go:** Allowing your child to lead their life is one of the most significant challenges of this transition. It's natural to worry, but trust in the values and lessons you've instilled in them.
- **Shifting from director to advisor:** Embrace a new perspective on parenting. Instead of directing their every move, become an advisor. Offer guidance when asked, but let them make their decisions and learn from them.

In this chapter, we've explored the incredible journey of watching our children transition from teenagers into adults and the psychological changes that both they and we must adapt to. It's a period filled with uncertainty, adjustments, and new dynamics, but it's also a time of growth, discovery, and opportunities for deeper connection.

I've shared stories, struggles, and insights and delved into expert opinions and research-backed information to help us understand this crucial phase in our children's lives. We've learned that our adult children are on a quest for independence, self-discovery, and defining their own identities. They might push boundaries, question our guidance, and even challenge our beliefs. It can be tough, but remember, it's all part of their journey to becoming self-sufficient, responsible adults.

As we move into the next chapter, we'll focus on reconnecting and repairing our relationships with our adult children. It's time to build bridges, rebuild trust if needed, and foster a sense of mutual respect and understanding. We'll look into practical strategies and conflict resolution tips for nurturing bonds that last a lifetime.

Chapter 5:
Reconnecting, Rebuilding, and Strengthening Relationships With Adult Children

I have always believed that the most precious thing in life is the bond we share with our children. As a mother of two wonderful young adults, I've had my fair share of challenges and joys in navigating the transition from parenting children to parenting adults.

In this chapter, we will delve into the delicate yet transformative process of reconnecting, rebuilding, and strengthening our relationships with our adult children. It's not uncommon for the once-close bonds we had with them to feel strained or even estranged as they embark on their own life paths. The heartache and frustration that can come with this territory can feel insurmountable but I also know that there's hope, healing, and growth on the horizon.

Throughout this chapter, we will explore practical strategies and real-life examples to help you navigate the often treacherous waters of reconnecting with your adult children. We will delve into the complexities of resolving conflicts, setting healthy boundaries, and finding common ground. It's about fostering an environment where both you and your children feel heard, respected, and valued, even as they spread their wings and fly.

You'll hear stories from parents who have faced similar challenges and triumphed. We'll also discuss the importance of self-reflection and personal growth as we adapt to our changing roles. It's not about being a perfect parent; it's about being a parent who is willing to grow, learn, and adapt to the ever-evolving landscape of parenthood.

So, let's roll up our sleeves, open our hearts, and explore how we can mend, rebuild, and strengthen the bonds with our adult children. It's a journey that promises growth, understanding, and the possibility of a deeper, more meaningful connection with the ones we love most.

Estrangement

Estrangement is a topic that no parent ever wants to think about, let alone experience. Yet, it's a reality that many of us may face at some point in our lives. Estrangement, in its simplest terms, is when adult children choose to cut off or limit contact with their parents, even when parents believe they have done nothing wrong. It's a heart-wrenching and confusing experience that can leave us feeling lost, hurt, and bewildered. But remember, you are not alone, and there is hope for healing and reconciliation.

To shed some light on this topic, let me share the story of Louann and her daughter, Brenna. Their story may resonate with some of you, and it highlights the complexities of family dynamics in adulthood.

Louann and Brenna were once incredibly close. Their bond was unbreakable, and they could never have imagined that they would find themselves on the path of estrangement. Things started to change when Brenna got married. Before the wedding, Louann and her husband had been actively involved in helping to provide for Brenna and her son. But as Brenna embarked on this new chapter of her life, differences in parenting philosophies began to emerge between mother and daughter.

These disagreements may have seemed insignificant at first, but they gradually grew in intensity. Louann and Brenna struggled to find common ground, and as tensions simmered, their once-solid relationship began to unravel. The breaking point came when Brenna made the painful decision to tell her mother that she would no longer allow her to see her grandson. Louann was utterly devastated by this ultimatum.

In the face of this heartbreaking situation, Louann wanted answers. She desperately wanted to mend their fractured relationship. However, Brenna's response was not what Louann had hoped for. Brenna refused to address the underlying issues or engage in an honest conversation about their past hurts. She asked for time. The divide between them only widened, and the pain of estrangement deepened.

Louann's story may resonate with many of you who have found yourselves in a similar situation. You may be wondering why adult children choose to cut off their parents, even when parents believe they have done nothing wrong. The reasons can be multifaceted and complex. Adult children may feel that their boundaries were not respected, that they weren't heard, or that their independence was stifled. Sometimes, past conflicts or unresolved issues can fester beneath the surface, causing a sense of resentment and frustration to build over time.

It's important to understand that estrangement often results from a culmination of issues and feelings rather than a single event. While it may be difficult to accept, our children are their own individuals, with their own beliefs, values, and experiences. As parents, we need to respect their autonomy and recognize that our role in their lives evolves as they grow into adulthood.

So, if you find yourself in a situation similar to Louann's, where your adult child has chosen to cut off contact, what can you do to move forward and potentially rebuild the relationship?

Resolving Conflicts With Adult Children

Rebuilding a relationship with your estranged adult children is a journey filled with hope, challenges, and opportunities for growth. It starts with you, the parent, taking the initiative to mend what's broken, even if you're not sure where to begin.

Initiate Change

Remember, your ultimate goal is not to prove who was right or wrong but to reconcile and restore the relationship. This journey begins with you taking the first step toward reconnection. Let's take a moment to reflect back on personality types. Is your adult child perhaps an (I) Introversion personality type? If so, you taking the step to initiate change would be most beneficial. If you recall, they are most likely to have a fear of vulnerability or rejection, and they often struggle with communication skills. By you starting the conversation, you give them the ability to reconnect more easily.

In the story above, Louann realized that some of her comments to her daughter, Brenna, had not been well-received. She had been critical and reacted without considering the impact of her words on her daughter. In an act of humility and vulnerability, Louann wrote a heartfelt letter to Brenna, asking for forgiveness and affirming her child for who she was.

At first, Louann faced the painful silence from Brenna. However, the letter played a vital role in conveying to her daughter that Louann wanted the relationship to heal and that she valued her daughter above their disagreements. Louann had to let go of her preconceived notions of disrespect or entitlement and instead focus on recognizing where her daughter was growing. This shift in perspective became the cornerstone of their journey toward reconciliation.

Apologize Sincerely

If you've identified specific mistakes you've made, offer a sincere apology. Take responsibility for your actions without making excuses. Your adult child needs to see that you acknowledge your errors and genuinely regret any hurt you may have caused. Louann acknowledged she was wrong for trying to tell Brenna how to parent her child. She owned her mistake and said she was sorry for not trusting her daughter's choices as a mother.

Be Humble

To rebuild a relationship with an estranged adult child, it's essential to move forward with humility, putting the relationship itself above all else. When approaching your child, avoid the defensive stance of trying to prove that you were right all along. Instead, extend yourself toward them and actively listen to their thoughts and feelings.

Acknowledge that, as parents, we don't always get things right, even when our intentions are rooted in love. Try to step back and see the bigger picture. Own up to your mistakes and be willing to say them out loud. For instance, Louann bravely apologized to her daughter for her controlling behavior and asked for forgiveness.

It's vital that you let your adult child know that you're aware of your past mistakes and are committed to changing your behavior. When you do this, you create an environment in which your child feels secure expressing themselves without fear of judgment.

Respect Boundaries

If your adult child has set boundaries, respect them. Boundaries are a way for them to feel safe and in control. Honoring their boundaries demonstrates your commitment to rebuilding trust. I understand this one can be tough. All you want to do is reach out and hug them and wish for things to be the way they were. This can backfire, as it can be seen as controlling and smothering. Allow your adult child the space and respect they need during this time.

Find Common Ground

Rebuilding a relationship doesn't mean you and your adult child have to agree on everything. You may have differing perspectives on various issues, but that doesn't have to hinder your connection. Find common ground elsewhere. Your role as a parent is to provide support and love, not to control or dictate your child's choices. Louann and Brenna may never agree on parenting styles, but that doesn't mean they don't have other things in common.

Let go of any idealized expectations you may have had for your child's life. They are adults now, capable of mapping out their own future. Practice active listening and be open to their thoughts and ideas. Listen to what they say; you just might hear a point of view you never even considered. By focusing on what you can agree on and respecting their autonomy, you can begin the process of rebuilding trust.

Choose Affirmation

Even when your adult children make choices that you may not agree with, remember that they are still looking to you for acceptance and validation. Lay aside your opinions temporarily and meet your adult children where they are. Convey through your words and actions that you see them as whole individuals and that you love them deeply.

Louann made sure to tell her daughter that, despite their differences, she was there to support and love her. She knew that Brenna would make an amazing mother, and she was excited to watch her flourish.

Affirmation is a powerful tool for healing and reconciliation. By letting your adult child know that you respect their choices and value them as individuals, you create a foundation for rebuilding the relationship. Remember when we spoke of love languages? Is your child's love language affirmation? If so, this tool is perfect. They will feel loved, supported, and validated each time they hear those words of affirmation from you.

Let Go of Control

Louann's experience taught us the importance of respecting boundaries when trying to rebuild a relationship. If your adult child has requested space, honor that request. Take a step back and refrain from pushing or smothering them with unwanted communication.

When your child does reach out, remember to listen more than you speak. Your opinions may have already been communicated, and now it's their turn to express their thoughts and feelings without fear of judgment. By demonstrating respect for their boundaries, you can create an environment where they feel safe to share.

Take the Time Needed

Reconciliation and rebuilding trust take time, often longer than we would like. Every parent–child relationship is unique, and there's no easy solution. Be patient and don't rush the process.

Louann's journey with Brenna serves as a reminder that healing can be a slow and gradual process. It is normal to make some progress and then feel like there is no movement at all. There can also be backward movement on occasion. Small interactions can pave the way for positive communication. You may find that reminiscing about good memories or engaging in activities of mutual interest can help rebuild trust and connection.

Moving Forward After a Family Estrangement

Empowering your adult children to make their own choices and even allowing them to make mistakes is essential for their growth. Remember that they are still learning and evolving into their identities.

Instead of dwelling on their shortcomings or insisting on change, focus on moving forward in your relationship. By doing so, you model healthy communication and reaffirm your unwavering love for them.

Seek Professional Help

In some cases, it may be beneficial to involve a neutral third party, such as a therapist or counselor, to facilitate communication and provide guidance. A trained professional can help both parties navigate their emotions and work toward reconciliation.

While the path to rebuilding a relationship with an estranged adult child may seem daunting, it is a journey well worth embarking on. Keep the lines of communication open, maintain an open heart, and be prepared to embrace change.

Remember, every step you take toward reconciliation is a step closer to healing, and you are not alone on this journey. Countless parents have faced similar challenges and successfully reconnected with their adult children. Your love, patience, and commitment to the relationship can be a powerful force for positive change.

Strengthening Relationships

Nurturing bonds that last a lifetime with adult children after estrangement can be a delicate and challenging process. Here are some practical tips to help you reconnect and build a stronger, healthier relationship:

- **Self-reflection and accountability:** Begin by reflecting on your role in the estrangement. Take responsibility for any actions or behaviors that may have contributed to the rift. Acknowledge any mistakes or misunderstandings.

- **Open and honest communication:** Initiate a conversation with your adult child, expressing your desire to reconnect. Be open and honest about your feelings and willingness to work on the relationship. Avoid blame or defensiveness.

- **Active listening:** When your adult child is ready to talk, actively listen without interrupting. Validate their feelings and perspective, even if you don't agree. Show empathy and understanding.

- **Apologize and forgive:** If you deem it appropriate, apologize sincerely for any specific actions or behaviors that caused hurt. Be genuine in your remorse. At the same time, be willing to forgive any wrongs committed by your adult child. Forgiveness is a powerful healing tool.

- **Defining personal boundaries:** As you rebuild the relationship, establish clear and healthy boundaries that respect both parties' needs and feelings. Discuss and agree on what behaviors are acceptable and unacceptable.

- **Focus on the present and future:** Avoid dwelling on past grievances or conflicts. Instead, focus on building a positive and fulfilling relationship moving forward. Discuss shared goals, interests, and future plans.

- **Show consistency and reliability:** Demonstrate your commitment to the relationship by being consistent and reliable. Keep your promises and be there when your adult child needs you, showing that you are dependable and trustworthy.

- **Express unconditional love:** Remind your adult child that your love for them is unconditional. Regardless of past conflicts or estrangements, let them know that you love and care for them deeply. Do you recall your child's love language? We took a look at these in Chapter 2, giving us the ability to understand the best way we both give and accept love. Knowing the best way your adult child receives love will ensure they get this message loud and clear.

I've Tried Everything

One of the most painful things we can experience as a parent is losing contact with our adult child due to estrangement. It is grief. We feel the same pain that a loss brings. We yearn for their presence in our life.

Chloe's Story

Chloe is a vibrant 50-year-old mom of many, as she likes to say. All of her children are grown and she has spent significant time focusing on reinventing herself. For 25 years of her life, she gave all of herself to being "mommy." The day she was blessed with her first child, her life changed.

"My heart exploded, and no feeling has come close since." There would be times over the years that Chloe would have difficulty separating herself from them. The first day of school, sleepovers, summer camp, and that dreaded day they would move out on their own. She recalls driving her daughter to college and breaking out in hives.

"I am one of the lucky ones; my kids are my best friends. We get along so well and enjoy spending time together. We travel together once a year and talk every day."

Her oldest, a girl, would find herself in a relationship with a man the family would term "odd," and Chloe tried her best to engage with him. She immediately noticed how he was alienating her daughter from friends, and then family. Her once social, vibrant daughter, now dark and introverted. "Anytime I called her up to schedule time together, there was an excuse, but I could hear pain in her voice." Chloe said.

Chloe knew her daughter was covering up her pain. The more she pressed, the more tension would form between them. This would go on for years, until the couple would wed. The wedding would only be attended by ten people—none of his family or friends. Again, odd, right?

One year after the wedding, Chloe insisted her daughter come spend the weekend. She was worried about her drastic weight loss and reclusiveness. It would be her new son-in-law who would call and tell Chloe that he was putting distance between the two of them. He insisted that Chloe was not allowing her daughter to have a life of her own. The harder Chloe pushed back, the further away her daughter got.

She would spend sleepless nights sobbing, missing her daughter so much. Filled with worry, asking friends and family if they knew how she was doing. Each time she reached out, she was met with hostility or silence. She finally went to see a therapist for some help. It was then that she got some advice. She was reluctant to follow it at first, but it ultimately led to a reconciliation with her daughter.

As Chloe sat down across from her therapist, the first thing she was told to do was reach out one last time. With her jaw almost hitting the floor, shaking her head no, the therapist explained further. "I need you to reach out and tell your daughter that you are going to give her space. Let her know that you are there for support and unconditional love whenever she needs you."

Chloe was told to write this in a letter and send it, and then cease contact. It was the hardest thing she had ever had to do. Her therapist went on to explain that, in order to reconcile, there are a few things to consider:

- Always approach all situations lightly.
- It is best to handwrite a letter rather than speak because it gives you an opportunity to express your thoughts and feelings without interruptions.
- Be authentic in your words; this is not a time for name-calling or finger-pointing.
- Avoid big explanations or reiterating the past. Everyone is aware of the situation.
- Don't plead your case. State the facts and keep it brief.
- Apologize if you did anything wrong.
- Tell your child you are there for support and unconditional love.
- End the letter with a statement that you will be giving them space to allow them to make their own decisions. Avoid telling them you need space; this part should pertain to them.
- End with Love, Mom or Dad, making it simple and not open-ended.

Chloe followed these instructions explicitly and then heard nothing for over a year. She grieved that relationship with her daughter every day. She kept busy on days she wanted to call or show up. She allowed herself to have all the emotions, but she did not contact her.

She would hear from her daughter again, exactly when her daughter needed her. It had worked. Her daughter traveled that journey, made life decisions, and found her mother again.

It is important to understand that not all estrangements end this way. We often can find ourselves estranged and never have it resolved. We need to take care of ourselves. Talk to friends and family about how you are feeling. Talk to a therapist and make sure you are working through your emotions.

Remember that reconciliation and rebuilding trust may take time, and success is not guaranteed. It's important to approach the process with patience, empathy, and a genuine desire to heal the relationship. Keep in mind that the goal is not just to reconnect but to create a healthier and more meaningful bond that can truly last a lifetime. Next up is the art of communication. As parents, we have spent years talking to our children one way. Things change as they do, and communication is one of them.

Chapter 6:

How to Communicate With Adult Children

Communication is the cornerstone of any healthy relationship, and that includes the one we share with our grown-up sons and daughters. As parents, we've started down this path of raising our children, guiding them through the twists and turns of life, and watching them evolve into independent adults. Now, it's time to navigate a new phase, one where our role as parents shifts from being the primary decision-makers to being trusted advisors and, most importantly, loving supporters.

In this chapter, we're going to explore the art of communication with our adult children—a terrain that's often filled with challenges but equally brimming with opportunities for growth, connection, and lasting bonds.

As parents, we must recognize that our relationship with our adult children is not a static one. It evolves and transforms as they carve their own path in the world, just as we did in our time. The world they face today is vastly different from the one we encountered during our own formative years, and understanding these changes is essential to fostering healthy communication.

Throughout this chapter, you'll find real-life examples that illuminate the joys and challenges of communicating with adult children. You'll also gain insights from experts and research-backed information to help you navigate this terrain with confidence and grace. At the end of this chapter, you will find a questionnaire, the goal of which is to gauge how you feel you are doing in areas of communication, growth, connection, listening, coping, and self-reflection. It aims to offer you insights into what areas you are doing well and where you could focus more attention.

So, if you're ready to explore how to communicate effectively with your adult children, let's start together. By the end of this chapter, you'll be armed with practical strategies and a renewed sense of confidence to navigate the shifting sands of communication and maintain the precious connection you share with your adult children.

Let's dive in and discover the keys to strengthening the bonds that matter most.

Communicating With Our Adult Children Effectively

Practice Active Listening: A Powerful Form of Respect

One of the cornerstones of effective communication with adult children is the art of active listening. It's a skill that requires patience, empathy, and a genuine willingness to understand their thoughts and feelings.

Active listening involves more than just hearing words; it's about genuinely understanding what your adult child is trying to communicate. Here's how you can practice it:

- **Give them your full attention:** When your child wants to talk, put aside distractions like phones or TV. Show them that they have your undivided attention. This simple act sends a powerful message of respect.

- **Empathize and validate:** Try to see the situation from their perspective. Even if you don't agree with their point of view, acknowledging their feelings and experiences validates their emotions. For example, you could say, "I can understand why that would be frustrating for you." Do you have an adult child who uses emotional support as a coping strategy? Then this is a big one for you. Your child will be seeking comfort, understanding, and connection from you during challenging or emotionally distressing times.

- **Ask open-ended questions:** Encourage them to express themselves by asking open-ended questions like, "Can you tell me more about how you're feeling?" This shows that you are genuinely interested in what they have to say. Do you remember when we discussed personality types? If your adult child is an NT or an analyst, they often struggle to express their emotions. They are very brain-focused and need time to process. When you give them tangible questions, they feel more in their element.

- **Avoid jumping to solutions:** As parents, our natural instinct is to protect and solve problems for our children. However, sometimes they just need a sounding board. Instead of immediately offering solutions, ask if they want advice or simply someone to talk to. If your child uses emotional expression as a coping strategy, this is vital for them. When they vent, they seek emotional relief and validation for their experiences. In such cases, empathizing with and validating their emotions, instead of just solving their problems, become crucial components in improving the parent-child relationship.

- **Respect their personal space:** It's essential to respect their boundaries when they need space or don't want to discuss a particular topic. Pushing too hard can lead to strained relationships.

Let me share a personal story to illustrate the power of active listening.

Sasha's daughter, Emily, moved to a new city for a job opportunity. She was excited but also scared. Initially, she couldn't help but give her advice about where to live, how to budget, and so on. However, she soon realized that Emily needed her to listen more than to guide. So, during one of their phone calls, she asked, "Emily, how are you feeling about this big move?" That opened the floodgates, and Emily shared her excitement, fears, and hopes. She listened, empathized, and resisted the urge to offer solutions. Over time, their relationship deepened because Emily knew she was there to support her, no matter what. Their communication became more open, honest, and respectful.

Emotional Intelligence in Parenting Adult Children

Let's start by recognizing that our adult children are no longer the little ones we could easily guide and protect. They've grown into independent people with their own thoughts, feelings, and life paths. As parents, it's important to communicate with emotional intelligence, understanding their perspectives and fostering an open, respectful dialogue.

- **Avoid guilt tripping or emotional manipulation:** Remember, guilt trips and emotional manipulation can harm your relationship with your adult child. This can lead to your child adopting behavioral disengagement because they find interaction with the parent emotionally exhausting. Instead, focus on expressing your feelings and concerns honestly without resorting to tactics that make them feel guilty or manipulated. For example, instead of saying, "You never call me anymore, and I'm so lonely," try saying, "I miss our conversations and would love to hear how you've been."

- **Avoid using money as a control tool:** Money can be a powerful tool, but using it to control or manipulate your adult child's decisions can lead to resentment and strained relationships. While it's okay to help financially when needed, it's essential to maintain boundaries and avoid making your support conditional. Encourage financial independence and have open discussions about money, boundaries, and expectations.

- **Forgive yourself and your adult children for mistakes:** Mistakes are a part of life, and that includes our interactions with our adult children. Don't be too hard on yourself or them when misunderstandings or conflicts arise. It's perfectly normal for differences to surface, but forgiveness and understanding can go a long way in maintaining a healthy relationship. Remember, we're all learning and growing, even as parents.

Amanda and Robert have a son, Alex, who made a significant career decision that they didn't agree with. Their initial reaction was to push him to reconsider, even resorting to emotional manipulation by expressing how disappointed they felt. It only pushed him further away. When they realized their mistake, they apologized and genuinely listened to his reasons. They found common ground and strengthened their bond through open communication.

Research consistently shows that emotionally intelligent parenting leads to better relationships with adult children. By practicing empathy, active listening, and respecting their autonomy, we can create an environment where they feel understood and valued (**Sánchez-Núñez et al., 2020**).

Dr. Ellen Hendriksen, a clinical psychologist, advises, "In your interactions with adult children, prioritize understanding over control. Validate their emotions and experiences, even if you don't always agree with their choices. Building trust through open, non-judgmental communication is crucial" (**Hendriksen, 2019**).

Handling Conflicts Between Siblings in Adulthood

It's not uncommon for sibling conflicts to persist into adulthood and sometimes even intensify. It's essential to remember that your role as a parent now shifts more toward being a mediator and a supporter rather than a referee. It is important to remember the three core beings of your children when conflict arises. Love language, personality type, and coping strategy. Your children will have conflict because these will vary among them. When they try to work through things, keeping these in mind will be beneficial. If your oldest child needs validation but your youngest needs affirmation, be mindful of that. If your middle child expresses themselves with emotion, but your oldest uses avoidance and would rather not deal with any of the issues, you can see how conflict would arise. Have an open conversation with them as well and point out these differences. It could go a long way in helping. Here are some strategies to navigate sibling conflicts in adulthood:

- **Open communication:** Encourage your adult children to talk openly and honestly with each other. Create a safe space where they can express their feelings and concerns without fear of judgment. Your role here is to listen actively and validate their feelings.

- **Stay neutral:** Avoid taking sides in conflicts between your adult children. It's essential to remain neutral and not contribute to the tension. Your goal is to help them find common ground and resolve their issues independently.

- **Set boundaries:** While you want to be a source of support, it's important to set boundaries and not get overly involved in their conflicts. Let them take ownership of their issues and learn to resolve them as adults.

- **Encourage empathy:** Encourage your children to put themselves in each other's shoes. Help them understand each other's perspectives and feelings. Sometimes, a little empathy can go a long way in resolving conflicts.

- **Offer guidance when asked:** If your adult children seek your advice or guidance, be ready to provide it. However, make it clear that you're there to help, not dictate solutions. Offer suggestions, but let them make their own decisions.

Remember, conflicts between siblings can be challenging, but they can also be an opportunity for growth and strengthening relationships. By being a supportive presence and facilitating open communication, you can help your adult children navigate these conflicts successfully.

Negotiating Care for Elderly Parents Alongside Siblings

As parents age, the responsibility of caregiving may fall on the shoulders of your adult children and their siblings. Negotiating care for elderly parents can be a complex and emotionally charged process, but it's essential to work together. Here's how to approach it:

- **Start early:** Begin discussing your future care needs with your children before they become critical. Having these conversations early can help prevent misunderstandings and conflicts later on.

- **Hold family meetings:** Regular family meetings can be a valuable tool for discussing caregiving responsibilities. Everyone can share their thoughts and concerns, and you can collectively come up with a plan.

- **Determine roles and responsibilities:** Clearly define each child's role and responsibilities in caregiving. Consider each person's strengths, availability, and resources when assigning tasks. This will cause less conflict among siblings if you are no longer able to make decisions for yourself.

- **Seek professional advice:** Consult with professionals, such as financial advisors, geriatric care managers, or elder law attorneys, to help you make informed decisions about your care and financial matters.

- **Stay flexible:** Be prepared to adapt your caregiving plan as your needs change. Flexibility and open communication are key to successful caregiving collaboration.

- **Take care of yourself:** Remember that caregiving can be emotionally and physically draining. Talk now with your children about the importance of their well-being, and encourage them to take care of themselves along the way.

As we all know, keeping the lines of communication open with our grown-up sons and daughters can be a bit tricky. The dynamics have shifted, and it's essential to adapt our approach to maintain healthy, meaningful connections.

Keeping the Conversation Flowing

I've found that being empathetic, understanding, and supportive can go a long way in building trust and keeping the conversation flowing. So, let's discuss some examples of conversation starters, and I'll also share a few open dialogue strategies to foster those all-important healthy communication patterns.

Conversation starters:

- **"I'd love to hear about what's been going on in your life lately. Anything exciting or challenging you want to share?"**

  Starting with a genuine interest in your child's life is a great way to show that you care and are available for meaningful conversations.

- **"Is there something on your mind that you'd like to talk about? I'm here to listen and support you."**

  This open-ended invitation lets them know you're ready to engage in any topic that matters to them.

- **"I was thinking about our family vacation when you were younger. What are some of your favorite memories from those times?"**

  Reflecting on shared experiences can spark nostalgia and open up opportunities to reminisce about cherished moments.

- **"I read an article about [a topic of their interest] recently. Have you heard about it? I'd love to get your perspective."**

  Showing curiosity about their interests and opinions demonstrates that you value their knowledge and insights.

- **"I've been trying to learn more about [a topic they're passionate about]. Can you recommend any books or resources?"**

  This not only fosters a connection but also allows you to grow together through shared interests.

Open Dialogues: Fostering Healthy Communication Patterns

Now that we've covered some conversation starters, let's explore strategies to maintain open dialogue with your adult children:

- **Respect boundaries:** Acknowledge that your children have their own lives and responsibilities. Respect their time and space, and don't push them to share more than they're comfortable with.

- **Avoid judgment:** Be nonjudgmental and open-minded, even if you disagree with their choices. Remember, they are adults capable of making their own decisions.

- **Regular check-ins:** Make an effort to check in regularly, but not excessively. A casual text or call to ask how they're doing can go a long way in maintaining a connection.

- **Share your life:** Don't hesitate to share your own experiences and challenges. This can create a sense of reciprocity in the relationship.

- **Ask for advice:** As your child grows, ask them for advice on things you are struggling with, whether it is a decision about an upcoming work project or a difficult coworker. If you ask for their input, they will feel valued and that you respect their opinion.

Remember, communication is a two-way street. Sometimes it might take time for your children to open up or adjust to these new dynamics. Patience and consistency are key.

How Modern Technology Affects Communication

In this age of rapid technological advancement, our lives have been profoundly impacted by the digital revolution. We've witnessed the younger generation effortlessly adapt to the digital world while we sometimes struggle to keep up. Our children, whether they're in their twenties or thirties, are natives in this digital landscape, and as parents, we need to understand how technology is shaping our relationships with them.

I'm sure many of you have seen those adorable videos of babies trying to interact with magazines, swiping and tapping, as if the world has always been a touch screen. It's a testament to how deeply technology has permeated our lives, and it's not just the young ones.

Erin has a grandfather who just celebrated his 87th birthday. Three years ago, when she lost her grandmother, he couldn't even operate the washing machine. Yet, now, each Sunday, she is greeted with a FaceTime visit from him. He has welcomed technology into his life to stay connected to his loved ones.

The convenience of technology has been undeniable. It has softened the blow for many parents who send their children away to college or pack them off for their own adventure. Parents know they can still stay in touch and even see their faces anytime, day or night, which helps.

However, let's be honest; this level of connectivity can have its downsides. It's easy to become overly attached, and boundaries can get blurred. Adult children may feel overwhelmed when parents demand constant contact, whether it's daily check-ins, adding them on every social media platform, or even commenting publicly on their posts. It's crucial for us, as parents, to find a balance between staying connected and respecting their need for independence and growth.

Let's take a moment to explore the pros and cons of technology in our communication with our adult children:

The pros:

- **Staying connected:** Technology allows us to stay in touch with our children, no matter where they are in the world. Video calls, text messages, and social media make it easier than ever to bridge the physical gap.

- **Sharing moments:** Through photos, videos, and instant messaging, we can share important moments in our lives, and they can share theirs. It's a wonderful way to remain a part of each other's daily experiences.
- **Support and advice:** Technology makes it possible for us to be there for them when they need advice or support, even if it's just a phone call away. This can be especially reassuring during challenging times.
- **Education and awareness:** Technology can help us understand their world better. We can follow their interests, read about the issues that matter to them, and have more informed conversations.

The cons:

- **Invasion of privacy:** When we cross boundaries by demanding constant updates or commenting on their social media, we risk invading their privacy. It's important to remember that they are adults entitled to their own space.
- **Dependency:** Constant connectivity can create a dependency that may hinder their personal growth and independence. It's essential to encourage them to spread their wings.
- **Miscommunication:** Misunderstandings can arise from misinterpreted text messages or comments online. It's important to maintain open and honest communication to avoid unnecessary conflicts.
- **Distraction:** Technology can sometimes distract us from meaningful face-to-face interactions. Nothing is worse than feeling unheard because the person across from us is staring at their phone. Encourage quality time together without screens.

As we navigate this digital age, let's remember that technology can be a blessing and a curse when it comes to communicating with our adult children. The key is finding a balance that respects their autonomy while nurturing the connection we cherish. In the end, it's not about how often we connect but about the quality of those connections that truly matter.

My Advice Is Being Dismissed

One of the most challenging aspects of parenting adult children is communication. We've all been there—you're trying to offer advice or share your perspective, and it seems like your being ignored. It's frustrating, disheartening, and can leave you feeling powerless. But I'm here to tell you that you're not alone in experiencing this, and there are ways to navigate these tricky waters with grace and understanding.

First, it's important to acknowledge that our adult children are now independent people with their own thoughts, beliefs, and experiences. They are no longer the children who hung on to our every word, and that's a natural part of their growth and development. While it might feel like they're rejecting or dismissing your advice, it's more likely that they're asserting their independence.

So, what can we do when it seems like all our well-intentioned suggestions are being dismissed?

- **Tell them how you feel:** So often, we can begin to feel a certain way, and our adult children have no idea. We can't fix these things unless everyone is aware of the issue. Have a sincere chat about how you are feeling. What is it they are doing that is making you feel this way? Offer solid solutions. For example, your daughter calls you complaining about her husband. You suggest she take a weekend away and relax. She immediately interrupts you, claiming you don't understand, and hangs up. You need to tell her how this hurts your feelings, that you do have experience with this from your own marriage, and all you want to do is make sure she is okay.

- **Validate:** This is a two-way street. If your child is coming to you with an issue but slamming your suggestion in your face, you need to address it. For example, your son wants advice on how to deal with a difficult boss. You suggest that he request a meeting and prepare a list of things he is struggling with beforehand. Your son rolls his eyes, gets up, and, as he is leaving, says, "That's ridiculous." Validate that he is feeling frustrated, but be sure to validate your own feelings in this. Be sure he understands how his comment made you feel.

- **Avoid problem-solving:** Instead of jumping into problem-solving mode right away, offer your support and let them know you're there for them. Say something like, "I'm here to support you while you figure this out." This approach opens the door for them to figure it out on their own and leaves you to offer emotional support.

- **Give and take space:** Sometimes, we all need space. It's essential to respect those boundaries. If they're not receptive to your advice at the moment, let them know you're available when they are, and then give them the space they need. If you are feeling dismissed, voice your concerns and advise them that you need some space but will be there for support when needed.

- **Reflect:** Take a moment to contemplate your communication style. Are you coming across as judgmental or critical? Are you offering unsolicited advice? Being aware of your communication patterns can help you make adjustments that create a more open and receptive atmosphere.

Remember, the goal here is not to change your adult child's mind or make them follow your advice blindly. It's about fostering a healthy, respectful, and open line of communication.

When to Advise and When to Help

As our children grow into adulthood, it's natural for us to want to continue guiding and protecting them. After all, we've spent years nurturing them, and the instinct to offer advice is deeply ingrained. However, in this new phase of life, it's vital to approach this desire with a delicate touch. Here's how:

Avoid Unsolicited Advice

Think back to when you were their age. Did you appreciate unsolicited advice? Most likely not. Remember, our adult children are forging their own paths and making their own decisions. They might not always follow our guidance, and that's okay. Wait until they ask for advice before offering your wisdom. This shows respect for their autonomy and independence.

Broach the Topic Thoughtfully

When you sense they might benefit from your advice or guidance, approach the topic in a nonconfrontational or non-passive-aggressive manner. Find the right moment, and express your concern with love and understanding. Say something like, "I've been thinking about this, and I'd love to share my perspective if you're open to it."

Offer Help When Asked

Remember that offering help only when asked is a powerful way to foster self-reliance and resilience in your adult children. When they seek your assistance, it means they value your input and are more likely to take it to heart. This also builds trust in your relationship.

Don't Take Things Personally

Adult children, just like everyone else, have their good days and bad days. If they react with frustration or resistance when you offer advice or help, don't take it personally. Remember that emotions can run high, and it's not a reflection of your parenting or your intentions.

Let Them Learn from Mistakes

Mistakes are an essential part of personal growth and development. Instead of rushing in to fix things for them, give your adult children the space to learn from their own experiences. They'll become more self-sufficient and confident in their decision-making.

Learn to Let Go

This can be one of the toughest aspects of parenting adult children. Learning to let go means allowing them to make choices, even if they're different from what you'd prefer. Trust that they will make the best decisions for themselves, and be there to support them when they ask for it.

Trust in Your Values

Remember the values you instilled in them during their upbringing. Trust that those values will guide them, even when you're not around to offer guidance. Your influence is still present, shaping their choices and actions.

Give Advice Without Imposing

When you do offer advice, be mindful not to impose your views on them. Share your thoughts and experiences, but allow them the freedom to make their own decisions. Remember, it's their life to lead, and they need the space to do so.

Avoid Interfering in Personal Relationships

Respect their personal relationships and boundaries. While you may have opinions about their choices in friends or partners, it's essential to avoid interfering unless you genuinely believe there's a danger to their well-being.

How to Be Supportive When You Disagree

In this section, we'll explore how to maintain a strong, supportive connection with your adult children even when you don't see eye to eye on everything.

Love Is Unconditional: Approval Isn't

We need to understand that your love for your children is unwavering, but approval of their choices doesn't always come naturally. You may find yourself disagreeing with some of their decisions, and that's okay. Remember, it's their life to live, and they need the freedom to make their own choices, even if they make mistakes along the way. It's your role as a parent to provide guidance and support but not necessarily to dictate their path.

You Can Disagree Without Causing Conflict or Hurt

Creating an open and nonjudgmental space for discussions is essential. Let your adult children know that you value their opinions and are willing to listen, even when you disagree. Encourage them to express their thoughts and feelings without fear of condemnation, fostering a sense of mutual trust and respect.

Practice Patience

Patience is the key to maintaining a harmonious relationship. It's natural to have disagreements, but patience allows us to navigate these differences with understanding. Take a deep breath and remind yourself that it's okay for them to have their own perspectives, just as you do.

Be Positive and Optimistic When It Gets Tough

When disagreements arise, try to focus on the bigger picture—your love for each other and the strength of your relationship. Positivity and optimism can help defuse tense situations and keep communication lines open. Remember, it's possible to disagree and still maintain a loving and respectful connection.

Disagreements Are Normal; What Matters Is How You Handle Them

Disagreements are not a sign of a failing relationship; they are a natural part of any human interaction. What truly matters is how you handle these disagreements. Approach them with empathy, active listening, and a willingness to understand their perspective, even if you don't agree with it.

Always Be Their Safe Haven

One of the most beautiful aspects of parent–child relationships is the unshakable sense of security that parents can provide. Remind your adult children that you are there for them, no matter what life throws their way. Knowing they have your unwavering support can give them the courage to face challenges and make difficult choices.

Coping When You Disapprove

It's perfectly normal to have concerns about your child's lifestyle choices, but remember that your role now is more about guidance than control. Share your concerns respectfully, express your love, and offer your support without judgment. Ultimately, it's their life to lead, and they will learn from their own experiences.

How to Handle Sensitive Topics

Another critical part of communicating with our adult children is the area of sensitive topics. Let's explore how to handle those with grace and respect.

The first step in fostering strong communication with your adult children is to create an environment where they feel comfortable discussing sensitive topics. This means you need to be an active listener, open-minded, and nonjudgmental. When they know they can approach you without fear of criticism, it paves the way for healthy conversations.

Understand the Importance of Mental Health

In today's world, the importance of mental health is undeniable. Many young adults face stress, anxiety, and even depression. Encourage open and supportive conversations about the well-being of their mental health. Let them know you are there to support them, and it's okay to seek help when needed. Sharing your own experiences with mental health challenges, if applicable, can also break down barriers and normalize the conversation.

Guiding an Adult Child Through Career Decisions

Career decisions can be daunting, and your guidance can be invaluable. However, it's important to strike a balance between offering advice and allowing them to make their own choices. Share your insights and experiences, but remember, it's their path to forge. Be a sounding board rather than a decision-maker.

Helping Them Manage Their Finances Responsibly

Money matters can often be a touchy subject. When it comes to financial discussions, approach them with sensitivity. Share your knowledge about budgeting and financial responsibility, but refrain from imposing your views. Offer support without taking control. Remember, they're adults now, and their financial choices are ultimately theirs to make.

Family Problems

Family conflicts, past or present, may need to be addressed for closure or resolution. Ignoring them may be preferable for many, but breaking generational patterns and healing should take precedent. These conversations can be emotional and require empathy and understanding. Take the lead and be an example. Maybe begin the conversation by allowing your children to know about any work you have done to heal your own past.

Romantic Relationships

There will be many partners your children choose whom you won't approve of or like. They can choose people to share their lives with who we believe don't treat them well, respect them, or value them the way we think they deserve. Approach conversations about their romantic partners with sensitivity. Share your concerns if you have any, but ultimately respect their choices.

Difficult Conversations About Health, Aging, or End-of-Life Decisions

Conversations about health, aging, or end-of-life decisions are some of the toughest ones to broach. Approach these topics with the utmost care and compassion. Express your concerns and wishes, but respect their autonomy. It's about finding common ground and making decisions that reflect the values of everyone.

Adjusting to the Role of Grandparent

As your adult child becomes a parent themselves, you'll naturally step into the role of a grandparent. This transition can evoke a mix of excitement and challenges. Remember that your child is now the primary parent, and your role is supportive. Offer help when requested, respect their parenting choices, and cherish the moments you share with your grandchildren.

In the ever-changing landscape of parenthood, one thing remains constant: the need for open and respectful communication. Realize that these conversations might not always be easy, but they are essential. By fostering an environment of trust, empathy, and understanding, you can bridge the generation gap and maintain a strong bond with your adult children.

Self-Assessment Questionnaire

As I stated at the beginning of this chapter, I wanted to include this questionnaire as a way for you to gauge how you feel you are doing as a parent to an adult child. The goal is to assess your feelings and perceptions in various areas related to parenting. This questionnaire is designed to help you reflect on your strengths and areas for improvement in communication, growth, connection, listening, coping skills, and self-reflection as parents of adult children.

Please rate the following statements on a scale from 1 to 5, with 1 being "Strongly Disagree" and 5 being "Strongly Agree." Feel free to add comments or explanations as needed.

Communication

I feel that I effectively communicate with my adult children.

☐ (Strongly Disagree)

☐ (Disagree)

☐ (Neutral)

☐ (Agree)

☐ (Strongly Agree)

I am open to listening to my adult children's perspectives and ideas.

☐ (Strongly Disagree)

☐ (Disagree)

☐ (Neutral)

☐ (Agree)

☐ (Strongly Agree)

I encourage open and honest communication with my adult children.

☐ (Strongly Disagree)

☐ (Disagree)

☐ (Neutral)

☐ (Agree)

☐ (Strongly Agree)

Growth and Connection

I actively support my adult children's personal growth and development.

☐ (Strongly Disagree)

☐ (Disagree)

☐ (Neutral)

☐ (Agree)

☐ (Strongly Agree)

I feel connected to my adult children on both emotional and practical levels.

▢ (Strongly Disagree)

▢ (Disagree)

▢ (Neutral)

▢ (Agree)

▢ (Strongly Agree)

Listening

I actively listen to my adult children without judgment or interruption.

▢ (Strongly Disagree)

▢ (Disagree)

▢ (Neutral)

▢ (Agree)

▢ (Strongly Agree)

Coping Skills

I am able to handle conflicts and challenges with my adult children in a constructive manner.

☐ (Strongly Disagree)

☐ (Disagree)

☐ (Neutral)

☐ (Agree)

☐ (Strongly Agree)

Self-Reflection

I regularly take time to reflect on my parenting approach and make necessary adjustments.

☐ (Strongly Disagree)

☐ (Disagree)

☐ (Neutral)

☐ (Agree)

☐ (Strongly Agree)

I seek feedback from my adult children about my parenting and am willing to make changes based on their input.

▢ (Strongly Disagree)

▢ (Disagree)

▢ (Neutral)

▢ (Agree)

▢ (Strongly Agree)

Additional comments or insights:

Please provide any additional comments, thoughts, or insights you have about your parenting journey with your adult children.

Thank you for taking the time to complete this questionnaire. Your honest responses will help you gain valuable insights into your strengths and areas for improvement in your role as a parent of adult children.

We covered a lot of ground on the topic of communication in this chapter. The goal was to emphasize boundaries, respect, and a mutual understanding of active listening, empathy, and growth as we continue this journey with our adult children. Moving into the next chapter, we will explore the importance of boundaries. Our relationships can thrive if we know how to set and respect them. Let's jump in!

Chapter 7:

Boundaries—Knowing How to Set and Respect Them

Welcome to the next chapter of our journey together as we continue navigating the intricate waters of parenting adult offspring. We now come to a topic that is both important and delicate: setting and respecting boundaries. It's a subject close to my heart because, like you, I've had my share of challenges and triumphs in this area with my own son and daughter.

Boundaries are like the invisible fence lines that define the space between us and our adult children. They can be tricky to establish and maintain, but they are essential for nurturing healthy, evolving relationships with our grown-up offspring. Within these pages, we'll explore the art of setting boundaries with empathy and understanding, recognizing that our relationships with our children won't remain static and predictable.

Our aim isn't to impose rigid rules or to cling to outdated notions of authority, but rather to create a balance that respects both our children's autonomy and our own needs and values.

I want to offer you a safe space to explore the evolving dynamics of your relationship with your adult children. I understand that there will be moments of frustration and uncertainty, but also moments of joy, growth, and connection.

So, let's embark on this chapter together, with open hearts and a willingness to adapt to the changing landscape of parenthood. Together, we can learn how to set and respect boundaries in a way that strengthens our bonds with our adult children, creating a relationship that can thrive in this ever-evolving world.

Here's the thing: Have you ever wondered if you're caught up in a pattern of rescuing your adult child? Do you find it challenging to figure out where that line should be drawn between offering help and letting them stand on their own? If you do, you're not alone. Many of us grapple with this dilemma.

I once heard the saying, "It's easier to build a child than to repair an adult." We need to emphasize the importance of healthy boundaries between adult children and their parents. But, you know what? These boundaries must always come from a place of love, compassion, and respect. There is no doubt about it.

Now, let's talk about what those boundaries might look like in practice. Here are some examples:

- **Financial support:** You might set boundaries regarding financial assistance. Decide on a limit or specific purposes for the money you're willing to provide.

- **Living arrangements:** Boundaries about living arrangements can be important. You could discuss when and under what circumstances your adult child can live at home or contribute to household expenses if they choose to stay.

- **Privacy:** It's perfectly fine to establish privacy boundaries. Ask them to respect your personal space, set guidelines for accessing your rooms or belongings, or request advance notice for guests or parties at home.

- **Communication:** Boundaries around communication are vital. You can specify preferred methods of contact, how often you expect to hear from them, and the importance of respectful and considerate communication.

- **Personal choices:** When respecting their independence, express your expectations regarding specific behaviors, such as refraining from vaping in your presence, avoiding offensive language, and abstaining from illegal activities while living under your roof.

- **Mutual respect:** Establish boundaries centered on mutual respect. Set guidelines for conversations, emphasizing the importance of listening, avoiding judgment, and speaking kindly even during disagreements.

- **Time and availability:** Boundaries regarding your time and availability are crucial too. Specify when you're available for socializing, family events, or providing assistance, and communicate your need for personal time and space.

Remember, every family dynamic is unique, so the boundaries you set will depend on your individual circumstances and relationships. The key is open and respectful communication when discussing these boundaries with your adult children.

Now, I know it's not always a walk in the park, but here are some tips to help you maintain these healthy boundaries:

- **Recognize their adulthood:** Understanding that your child is now an adult is the foundational step. It means acknowledging that they have reached an age where they are entitled to make their own choices, decisions, and mistakes. Here's how to go about it:

    - **Autonomy and independence:** Embrace the fact that your adult child deserves autonomy and independence. Their life path may not mirror yours, and that's perfectly okay. Respect their right to choose their own direction, even if it differs from your expectations.

    - **Respect opinions and choices:** Your adult child has unique opinions, values, and dreams. Show genuine respect for their perspectives, even if they diverge from your own. Recognize that their choices are a reflection of their evolving identity.

    - **Lifestyle choices:** Whether it's their career, relationships, or personal beliefs, honor their lifestyle choices. Avoid imposing your views on them, and let them live in a way that feels authentic to them. Your role is now more about providing guidance when sought than dictating their choices.

- **Open communication:** Building effective communication is essential when building a healthy relationship with your adult child. It involves creating an environment where everyone feels heard, understood, and worthy. Here's how to make it work:
    - **Honest conversations:** Initiate open and honest conversations about boundaries. Share your thoughts, concerns, and expectations openly. Encourage your grown child to do likewise. Transparency is key. Keep in mind that if your child is an ISTJ (Introverted, Sensing, Thinking, Judging) personality type, this could be a struggle because they are fact-based and struggle with emotion. They prefer black-and-white rules as opposed to open-ended conversations that are subjective. They tend to be more reserved when discussing thoughts and feelings.
    - **Active listening:** Truly listen to what your child has to say. Understand their perspective, even if it differs from yours. Avoid interrupting or dismissing their feelings. Validating their emotions fosters trust and mutual understanding.
    - **Empathetic responses:** Respond with empathy and compassion. Acknowledge their feelings and emotions, even if you don't agree with their choices. Being empathetic helps bridge gaps and strengthens the parent–adult child connection.
- **Define your limits:** Setting and defining your boundaries is crucial for maintaining a healthy parent–adult child relationship. Here's how to effectively do it:
    - **Identify boundaries:** Take time to reflect on what you're comfortable with and what crosses the line for you. It could be about finances, personal space, time

commitments, or even emotional involvement. Identifying your boundaries is the first step.

  - **Consistency:** Once you've identified your limits, be firm and consistent in asserting them. Consistency helps your adult child understand your expectations and reduces confusion.

  - **Respectful communication:** When you communicate your boundaries, do so with respect and clarity. Avoid being confrontational or demanding. Frame your boundaries as a way to maintain a healthy and respectful relationship.

- **Respect and understanding:** Respecting your child's boundaries is as vital as setting your own. Here's how to achieve a balanced and respectful dynamic:

  - **Avoid Judgment:** Your adult child may have different needs, values, and priorities. Avoid being judgmental or critical of their choices. Accept that their path may lead them in directions you didn't anticipate.

  - **Finding Common Ground:** Strive to find common ground where both parties feel heard and respected. It's about compromise and understanding, rather than insisting on your way or theirs. Collaboration fosters stronger relationships.

- **Allow room for growth:** Setting boundaries is a learning process for both you and your adult child. Here's how to navigate this journey together:

  - **Mistakes Happen:** Understand that missteps may occur along the way. Be patient and forgiving when boundaries are crossed inadvertently. Use these moments as opportunities for growth and learning. If you have an adult child who uses avoidance as a coping strategy, this one may be difficult. They may prefer to avoid or ignore the mistake rather than discuss it, which will make them uncomfortable. They will want to avoid possible confrontations and fear your disappointment.

    - **Adaptability:** Be flexible and willing to adjust your boundaries as circumstances change. Growth and maturity can lead to evolving needs and expectations. Stay open to reassessing and adapting your boundaries as necessary.

- **Self-care:** Taking care of yourself is essential for maintaining your well-being and setting a positive example for your adult child. Here's how to prioritize self-care:

    - **Identify your needs:** Recognize your own needs and prioritize self-care to avoid becoming overwhelmed or resentful. When you prioritize self-care, you model the importance of self-respect for your adult child.

    - **Balanced lifestyle:** Strive for a balanced lifestyle that includes physical, emotional, and mental well-being. By upholding your boundaries and showing self-respect, you establish a model for your child to follow.

- **Seek professional help if needed:** Lean on professionals if you are struggling to build boundaries and maintain them or if issues with conflict persist. Here's how to approach this:

    - **Recognize the need:** If you're struggling to navigate complex family dynamics or feel that your efforts aren't yielding positive results, it's okay to seek help.

    - **Family therapist or counselor:** Reach out to a family therapist or counselor experienced in dealing with these issues. They can provide valuable insights, techniques, and a neutral perspective to facilitate productive discussions and solutions.

When Boundaries Are Not What They Seem

In some situations, adult children may use the need for "boundaries" as a pretext to maintain distance from their parents without entirely cutting them off. This approach might be chosen to avoid causing emotional distress to their parents while still establishing personal space and independence. Here's how parents can identify and address this situation:

Identifying the situation:

- **Lack of communication:** If adult children are setting strict boundaries without open communication about their reasons and feelings, it may indicate an issue.

- **Consistently evading:** If adult children consistently evade family events, gatherings, or conversations, citing boundaries as the reason, it may be a sign of distancing.

- **Emotional disconnection:** A noticeable emotional distance or avoidance of personal discussions can suggest that boundaries are being used to maintain distance.

What parents can do:

- **Open communication:** Start a conversation without judgment with your adult child. Try to understand their perspective and be willing to listen.

- **Respect their boundaries:** Acknowledge their need for personal space and boundaries, even if you don't fully understand or agree with them.

- **Express feelings:** Share your feelings and concerns calmly and respectfully. Let them know how their actions have affected you emotionally.

- **Seek compromise:** Explore ways to find a compromise that respects both their boundaries and your need for connection. Be open to adjustments that can meet both parties' needs.

- **Professional help:** If communication remains challenging, consider seeking the help of a family therapist or counselor to facilitate constructive dialogue.

It's essential for both parents and adult children to maintain a balance between individual autonomy and maintaining healthy family relationships. Understanding each other's perspectives and working together to find common ground can lead to more positive and harmonious interactions.

So, here's to fostering those healthy boundaries that nurture stronger, more fulfilling relationships with our adult children. Let's journey through this together with empathy, understanding, and a touch of humor because, hey, we're all in this together, right?

Chapter 8:

Empowering Autonomy—Nurturing Independence in Your Adult Child

In this chapter, we'll explore a topic that's close to the hearts of many parents: How to encourage independence in our adult children without inadvertently enabling them. I'll be sharing practical strategies and insights, drawn from real-life examples, to help you strike that delicate balance. We'll explore ways to support your adult child's journey to independence while steering clear of enabling behaviors that might hinder their growth.

You'll find stories from other parents who have been in your shoes, facing the same dilemmas and learning from their experiences. We'll build a sense of community and support because, trust me, you're not alone in this journey. We're all in this together, and together, we can help our adult children launch successfully into the world.

So, whether you're wondering how to encourage them to take responsibility for their finances, make their own career choices, or simply grow as individuals, this chapter will provide valuable insights and practical guidance to help you be the supportive, nurturing parent your adult child needs without crossing the line into enabling.

It's a natural instinct that never truly fades away. However, as our children transition into adulthood, our role in their lives needs to evolve, and it's crucial to understand the delicate balance between helping and enabling.

Times have changed, and the challenges they face are unique. Our role now isn't to hold their hands every step of the way but to empower them to stand on their own two feet. This process requires us to be both supportive and self-aware.

Understanding the Difference: Helping vs. Enabling

Helping and enabling are two sides of the same coin, and it's important to distinguish between them.

Helping

It involves offering assistance, guidance, and resources to enable your child to tackle challenges and make informed decisions. It empowers them to build essential life skills, learn from their mistakes, and grow into self-sufficient adults. Helping is about fostering independence by being a source of support rather than a crutch.

Enabling

This often stems from a well-intentioned desire to protect our children from pain or failure. However, it inadvertently fosters dependency and hinders their growth. Enabling typically involves doing things for your child that they should be doing for themselves, such as solving their problems, paying their bills, or making excuses for their mistakes.

Let me share a couple of real-life examples that might resonate with you.

Meet Alex, who has just graduated from college and is struggling to find a job. His mom, Lucy, has the means to support him financially, and her heart aches seeing her son stressed about bills and rent. When she offers temporary financial assistance to help him get on his feet, she is **helping**. However, continuously covering all his expenses and not encouraging him to actively seek employment is **enabling**.

Now, consider Mila, a talented artist who dreams of starting her own gallery. Her parents have concerns about the instability of the art world and discourage her from pursuing her passion. They think they are shielding her from the possibility of failure. In reality, they're **enabling** her to settle for a career she's not passionate about, rather than supporting her in pursuing her dreams.

Numerous experts agree on the importance of distinguishing between helping and enabling. Research shows that children who receive unconditional support and are allowed to face challenges independently tend to develop better problem-solving skills, resilience, and a stronger sense of self-worth. Conversely, enabling behavior can lead to learned helplessness, where children become reliant on their parents for even basic decisions (**Aikaterini Vasiou et al., 2023**).

Dr. Jane Nelsen, a renowned psychologist and author, suggests that parents should aim to be both "kind and firm." This means offering support and guidance while maintaining clear boundaries that encourage personal responsibility (**Next Step 4 ADHD, 20**20).

Navigating this shift in our parenting dynamic can be emotionally challenging. But remember, you're not alone on this journey. Many parents are facing the same uncertainties and dilemmas. Seek out support groups or engage with other parents who share your experiences. Sharing your stories, learning from others, and offering a listening ear can provide comfort and valuable insights.

In conclusion, our role as parents of adult children is not to shield them from life's hardships but to equip them with the tools they need to face those challenges head-on. Understanding the difference between helping and enabling is the first step toward fostering their independence and building a stronger, healthier relationship with them.

Financial Independence: When and How to Stop Financially Supporting Your Adult Children

One of the most significant milestones in your child's journey to independence is achieving financial self-sufficiency. While it's natural to want to continue supporting them, there comes a point when it's essential to stop enabling and allow them to help themselves. When is the appropriate time to cease providing financial support to our adult children?

- **Set clear expectations:** It's important to have open and honest conversations with your child about their financial independence. Discuss your expectations and timeline for them to become financially self-sufficient.

- **Gradual transition:** Instead of abruptly cutting off financial support, consider a gradual reduction. Encourage your child to take on more financial responsibility, such as paying for their rent, groceries, or insurance. Map out that timeline together and consider having them contribute while they are still living at home. Christine, a single mother of three, grew up with no financial guidance. It was always important to her to offer as much of this as she could to her own children. By age 16, she encouraged part-time jobs and summer employment. While they still lived at home, she had them open savings accounts. She taught them how to budget. By age 18, she had them pick three things they would be responsible for. Their cell phone bill, their self-care products, their entertainment—those types of things. If they chose to live at home into adulthood, it was important they contributed to bills. Once they left home, they would have an idea of how to pay bills and support themselves. They would be more prepared than she was, and she took comfort in that.

- **Offer guidance:** Help your child develop a budget, save, and invest wisely. Share your financial knowledge and offer advice when they seek it. Don't be afraid to share the mistakes you have made over the years. Many children are intimidated if their parents seem to have their finances sorted out. They can learn plenty from the things we got wrong and how we fixed them. Jamie and Michelle have twin sons, now 21. They never felt comfortable talking to their parents about money because they owned their own company and were quite successful. If the twins were having trouble making ends meet, they felt shame or embarrassment. When they communicated this to their parents, Jamie and Michelle started to talk about where they were financially at 21. This changed their relationship dynamic, and the boys were able to realize that they could also work toward a better financial future without judgment.

Supporting your child's financial self-sufficiency while considering their MBTI personality types and coping strategies can be highly effective. Here are some tailored approaches to consider:

For extroverted personality types (E):

- **Leverage networking:** Encourage them to utilize their social skills and networking abilities to explore job opportunities or find mentors in their field.

- **Teamwork:** Suggest collaborative financial strategies, such as group investments or shared living arrangements, that align with their preference for social interaction.

- **Public accountability:** Help them establish financial goals publicly, through social media or group challenges, to motivate them to stay on track.

For introverted personality types (I):

- **Independent research:** Support their preference for introspection by guiding them to research financial topics independently and make informed decisions.

- **Quiet budgeting:** Encourage them to create and manage a budget in a quiet, focused environment where they can reflect on their financial goals.

- **Savings habit:** Emphasize the importance of automating savings or investments, allowing them to grow their wealth without constant attention.

For sensing personality types (S):

- **Practical advice:** Provide concrete, step-by-step financial advice and tools to help them manage their finances in a practical and tangible way.

- **Short-term goals:** Focus on setting achievable short-term financial milestones that align with their preference for concrete, immediate results.

- **Hands-on learning:** Involve them in hands-on experiences, such as managing a small investment or starting a side business, to build financial skills.

For intuitive personality types (N):

- **Big-picture planning:** Encourage them to create a long-term financial vision and goals, aligning with their preference for conceptual thinking.

- **Investment in education:** Emphasize the value of continuous learning and skill development to enhance their earning potential over time.

- **Exploration:** Support their exploration of innovative financial strategies, such as investing in emerging technologies or startups.

For thinking personality types (T):

- **Analytical tools:** Provide financial analysis tools and resources that allow them to make logical and data-driven decisions.

- **Risk assessment:** Help them assess the risks and rewards of various financial choices, and encourage a balanced approach to investment and savings.

- **Budget automation:** Suggest using technology and automation to streamline budgeting and financial tracking.

Coping Strategies

- **Problem-solving copers:** If your child tends to use problem-solving coping strategies, engage them in discussions about financial challenges and work together to find practical solutions.

- **Emotion-focused copers:** For those who rely on emotion-focused coping, provide emotional support and understanding during financial setbacks, emphasizing that it's okay to seek help and express feelings.

Financially Supporting an Adult Child Without Enabling Them

Sometimes, your adult child may face financial difficulties, and it can be challenging to determine when to step in and help without enabling them. Here are a few tactics for achieving a balance:

- **Listen and empathize:** Begin by understanding their situation and listening without judgment. Express your support and willingness to help in a healthy way. Remind yourself that you were once young and may not have always had your finances sorted.

- **Offer non-financial support:** Sometimes, emotional support, guidance, or helping them explore alternative solutions can be more valuable than money.

- **Set boundaries:** Be clear about the extent of your financial assistance. Avoid enabling destructive behavior or creating dependency. Christine and Harry have five grown children. They like to be able to help them out financially when they need it. That being said, there is one hard and fast rule when it comes to money. If you borrow it, you must pay it back. They have taught their children that money is not a free resource in this world, and it should be treated with respect. As long as they pay it back under the terms they agree to, they are always welcome to borrow again if the time comes.

When to Stop Financially Assisting Adult Children

Knowing when to stop financially assisting your adult children can be emotionally challenging. Consider these factors:

- **Achieving financial milestones:** Look for signs of progress, such as them securing a stable job, paying bills consistently, and saving for their future. If they are doing well, it is time for a conversation.

- **Their comfort level:** Discuss with your child their comfort level with reducing financial assistance, and encourage them to take the lead in becoming financially independent.

- **Your own financial well-being:** Be mindful of your own financial health. Don't jeopardize your retirement or financial stability by continuing to support them excessively.

We also need to factor something else into this equation. What if our adult child adopts maladaptive coping strategies like distraction or denial? This could mean we find ourselves with a man child living in our basement, playing video games all day. We could end up with a daughter who sleeps until noon and spends her days lounging by the pool making Instagram stories. They are in complete denial about their financial situation and are living comfortably on our bank account.

If you find yourself in this situation, it is time to show that baby bird how to fly from the nest because those coping skills are now enabled, not helped, at this point.

There have been many parents who find themselves in a darker situation. They discover that their adult child has adopted substance abuse as a coping strategy. Instead of working toward their goals or finding that passion, their child is avoiding struggles under addiction. This is so difficult for parents, but the first step is going to be cutting off finances. Supplying the money for your adult child to continue to abuse any substance is enabling, not helping.

Coping With Feelings of Loss When Your Child Becomes Independent

Coping with the feelings of loss when your child becomes independent is a complex and emotional journey. It is important to reflect on and be mindful of your own coping strategy throughout this phase. It can be helpful when dealing with this loss. Lean into your own receiving love language as well. Let's dive deeper into this topic to provide you with more insights and strategies for managing these emotions.

Embracing the Evolving Relationship

When your child becomes independent, it's natural to experience a sense of loss. You might find yourself reminiscing about their childhood, missing the days when they depended on you for everything, and worrying about their well-being as they venture into the world on their own. However, it's important to recognize that this transition doesn't signify the end of your relationship with your child but rather its evolution.

Understanding the Grief Process

Just as with any significant life change, it's normal to go through a grieving process when your child becomes independent. Allow yourself all the time you need. You may have revolved your world around this child and are struggling to reinvent yourself. If you need help, don't hesitate to ask for it.

Finding Meaning and Purpose

One way to cope with feelings of loss is to find new meaning and purpose in your life. Consider exploring new hobbies, interests, or career opportunities that you may have put on hold while raising your children. By investing in your own personal growth and well-being, you can fill some of the void left by your child's newfound independence.

Staying Connected

While your child is becoming independent, it's essential to maintain a strong connection with them. Here are some ways to stay connected:

- **Meaningful conversations:** Continue to have open and honest conversations with your child about their life, experiences, dreams, and challenges. Display authentic curiosity in their thoughts and emotions. This is a great place to reflect on your receiving love language. If you need words of affirmation, this is what you should lean into with your adult child.

- **Visits and quality time:** Plan visits and spend quality time together. Whether it's a weekend getaway, a family dinner, or a holiday celebration, creating memorable moments can strengthen your bond.

- **Shared experiences:** Find common interests or activities that you can enjoy together. This could include hobbies, sports, or shared experiences like traveling or volunteering.

- **Digital communication:** In today's world, digital communication can bridge the physical gap. Video calls, texting, and social media can help you stay connected even if your child lives far away. Just remember those boundaries we discussed earlier.

Seek Support and Guidance

Don't hesitate to seek support from friends, family members, or support groups of parents going through similar transitions. Sharing your experiences and emotions with others who understand can be incredibly comforting and reassuring.

Embrace Your Child's Independence

Ultimately, the key to coping with feelings of loss when your child becomes independent is to embrace and celebrate their growth. Remember that your guidance and love have played a key role in preparing them for this stage of life. Your child's independence is a testament to your success as a parent. As they navigate the world on their own, take pride in the strong foundation you've provided them and have faith in their ability to thrive independently.

While the transition to your child's independence can evoke a sense of loss, it's important to recognize it as a natural part of the parenting journey. Embrace this evolution of your relationship and cherish the opportunities for continued connection and growth. With time, patience, and support, you can navigate this emotional transition and find joy in watching your child spread their wings and thrive in the world.

As we wrap up this chapter, I want to commend you on your commitment to learning and growing as a parent of adult children. Navigating the delicate balance between helping and enabling can be a challenging journey, but it's a journey worth taking.

It's essential to recognize that helping your adult child is a beautiful thing. Offering support, guidance, and love is what parents do. However, it's equally vital to discern when your assistance might be veering into enabling territory. Enabling can inadvertently hinder their growth and independence, which is not in their best interest.

As you move forward, remember that parenting is an evolving journey, and we're all learning together. In the next chapter, we'll delve into something equally important—celebrating your adult child's accomplishments. It's a joyful part of our ongoing relationship, and I'm excited to explore it with you.

Chapter 9:

Proud Parents—Celebrating the Accomplishments of Adult Children

Isn't it remarkable how quickly the years pass by? It seems like just yesterday we were guiding our kids through their first steps, teaching them to ride a bike, and helping with their homework. Yet here we are, with our children all grown up and navigating the world on their own. The journey of parenthood is an ever-evolving one, and as our children transition into adulthood, our roles shift as well. In this chapter, we will explore a topic that is both heartwarming and essential to maintaining healthy relationships with our adult children—celebrating their accomplishments.

In today's fast-paced and ever-changing world, it's vital for us as parents to recognize and celebrate our adult children's accomplishments. This goes beyond simply saying, "I'm proud of you." It involves understanding what these achievements mean to them, appreciating their individual journeys, and finding meaningful ways to show our love and support.

Throughout this chapter, we'll delve into practical strategies for expressing our pride and admiration for our adult children's accomplishments. We'll share real-life examples and personal stories to illustrate how different families have navigated this aspect of their relationships. We'll also draw on expert opinions and research-backed information to provide you with a comprehensive guide to celebrating your adult children's achievements.

So, let's celebrate the remarkable accomplishments of our adult children and ensure that they always know just how proud we are of them. In doing so, we can continue to nurture the beautiful relationship we share, adapting and growing alongside them as they journey into adulthood.

Why Do We Celebrate?

As a parent of adult children, I've come to realize the profound importance of celebrating their milestones and successes. Although it may be seen as self-indulgent or time-consuming at times, research has consistently demonstrated that celebrating significantly impacts our mental health, self-care, motivation, and happiness (***Why Celebrating*, 2021**). It's more than just a pat on the back we give ourselves or our adult children; it's a mindful practice that fills our lives in amazing ways.

Studies have consistently demonstrated the positive effects of celebrating accomplishments. It's more than just a fleeting moment of joy—it can lead to improved physical health and better coping strategies. When we take the time to reflect on and commemorate our successes, we tend to be more optimistic, take better care of ourselves, and experience lower stress levels. These benefits are universal, transcending socioeconomic factors, education, age, and gender (***Why Celebrating*, 2021**).

In the realm of positive psychology, there's a concept known as "savoring." It entails the process of noticing, appreciating, and enhancing positive experiences, such as celebrating our adult children's accomplishments. Savoring not only boosts our own feelings of self-worth but also contributes significantly to our overall life satisfaction. It expands our thoughts and behaviors, fosters creativity, strengthens social connections, enhances personal resources, and bolsters resilience. In essence, it's a holistic approach to well-being that enriches our lives and the lives of our loved ones.

By embracing the practice of celebration, we can strengthen our bonds with our grown-up children and find greater happiness and fulfillment in our lives.

Chuck and Michelle's Story

Proud parents of two grown children, a son, 29, and a daughter, 31. You will often hear these parents telling others just how different their children are. "Like night and day, I tell you, Mike is all tech and science, while Lucy is crazy about sports." Chuck said.

Raising the two of them has always been a balancing act. Michelle noticed quite early that her son was an introvert and needed extra time if schedules were going to change, and he thrived on routine. Her daughter, on the other hand, was easygoing and an extrovert. That being said, she was emotional and wore her heart on her sleeve. She could become frustrated or upset easily.

When it came to celebrating milestones for the children, they got a crash course in what worked and what didn't. Their daughter loved loud and colorful birthday parties. She would invite all of her friends and relish at the thought of attention. Their son emotionally melted during his one and only birthday party. He was too overstimulated and didn't care for the balloons or the number of people invading his space. He took refuge in his bedroom and only celebrated with family dinners from that year on.

Whether it came to school awards, tests, graduations, sports ceremonies, or tech conferences, each child grew into those same personalities. Their daughter, now 31, still enjoys sparkly shoes and pink birthday cake. Their son, a computer engineer, is most comfortable surrounded by those familiar to him. His ideal birthday celebration is his favorite dinner, ordered in.

As parents, Chuck and Michelle believed it was their job to adapt to their children's personalities to make sure they got the message across. "We love you, we support you, and we celebrate you. We meet you where you want to be met." They understood that this is how their children best heard them.

Never underestimate the power of expressing love and affection regularly. As our children grow into adulthood, they might not need our guidance in the same way as they did when they were younger, but they still need to know that our love for them remains unwavering. A simple "I love you" or a heartfelt hug can go a long way in assuring them that you're there for them, no matter what.

Encourage Them to Pursue Their Passions

Think about it like this: When your child was a toddler, you celebrated their every milestone, from their first steps to their first words. As adults, they're still achieving milestones, whether it's landing a new job, buying a first home, or simply managing the complexities of adult life. These accomplishments might not be as visibly dramatic as those early milestones, but they are just as significant. Celebrate them with the same enthusiasm and joy.

One of the most beautiful gifts we can give our adult children is the encouragement to pursue their passions. As they step into the adult world, they'll face numerous challenges and decisions. What they choose to pursue may not align with our own dreams or expectations for them, and that's perfectly okay. In fact, it's more than okay—it's essential.

Supporting their passions will not only lead to a more fulfilling life for them but also strengthen your relationship. Remember, we cannot expect our children to live out our unfulfilled dreams or follow a predetermined path. Instead, celebrate their unique interests and talents, even if they differ from your own.

Be Proud of Who They Are, Not Just What They Achieve

It's crucial to remember that our pride in our adult children should be rooted in who they are as individuals, not just in their achievements. While it's natural to take pride in their accomplishments, their worth as human beings goes far beyond what they do. Celebrate their character, their kindness, their resilience, and their uniqueness.

For instance, let's say your child is working a job that doesn't pay much, but they find immense satisfaction in their work because it aligns with their values. Instead of focusing solely on their income or job title, celebrate their dedication to making a positive impact. It's not about what they've achieved materially but about the values and principles they uphold.

As parents, we often fall into the trap of comparing our adult children's paths to our own or to the paths of others. It is also essential that you don't compare your children against one another. They are individuals and never need to hear, "Your brother is far more successful than you are." This may result in the adult child harboring resentment toward their parents or siblings. Additionally, the situation can worsen if the adult child employs maladaptive coping strategies such as self-blame, self-distraction, and behavioral disengagement.

Remember their strengths and what brings them joy will vary. It's important to remember that each person's journey is unique, and there is no easy formula for success or happiness.

Our role as parents is to provide support, guidance, and unwavering love as they navigate the complexities of adulthood.

How Do We Celebrate?

Let's dive into a few tips on how to do this effectively, and to make it even more relatable, I'll draw examples based on different MBTI personality types.

The ISTJ Child

Your ISTJ child values tradition and reliability. When they accomplish something, celebrate it in a traditional manner. Throw a small family dinner, bake their favorite cake, or frame their diploma. These gestures show them that you respect their accomplishments and are there to support them. If your adult child's love language is acts of service, this will also be effective.

The ENFP Child:

ENFPs are creative and spontaneous. Celebrate their accomplishments by joining in on their enthusiasm. Plan a surprise party or take them on an impromptu adventure. The key here is to match their energy and zest for life.

The INTJ Child

INTJs are analytical and focused. Celebrate their accomplishments by engaging in deep discussions about their achievements. Show genuine interest in their projects and ideas, and ask thoughtful questions. Your intellectual engagement will mean the world to them. This form of celebration is effective if your child also has the love language of quality time. They will appreciate the one-on-one time.

The ISFP Child

ISFPs are artistic and sensitive. Celebrate their accomplishments by creating a personalized gift or artwork that reflects their achievement. Take them to an art exhibition or a concert to honor their creativity. Keep in mind that if your child uses receiving gifts as their love language, they will resonate with this the most.

Boosting Self-Esteem and Confidence

Now, let's talk about boosting your adult child's self-esteem and confidence. This is an ongoing process that goes hand in hand with celebrating their accomplishments.

- **Active listening:** Show them that you genuinely care about their thoughts and feelings. Listen without judgment, and let them know their opinions matter.

- **Encourage independence:** Allow them to make their own decisions and learn from their mistakes. This autonomy helps them build confidence in their abilities.

- **Provide constructive feedback:** When they seek advice or guidance, offer constructive, noncritical feedback. Focus on their strengths and help them develop in areas they wish to improve.

- **Celebrate effort, not just results:** Highlight the effort they put into their endeavors, regardless of the outcome. This reinforces the importance of determination and hard work.

- **Set realistic expectations:** Avoid placing undue pressure on them. Understand their limitations and encourage them to set achievable goals.

Emma's Story

Emma's recently landed her dream job after years of hard work and dedication. She had faced five rejections, multiple tough interviews, and many moments of self-doubt, but she persevered. When Emma finally called her mom with the news, she couldn't have been prouder. They both cried, screamed, and talked about the future. They celebrated her accomplishment with a family dinner, and it was a beautiful reminder of how their roles as parents evolve.

Why is it important to continue to celebrate our adult children's accomplishments, you may ask? Well, here's why:

- **Validation and support:** When we celebrate our children's successes, big or small, we are letting them know that we see and appreciate their efforts. This validation strengthens their self-esteem and sense of self-worth.

- **Bonding:** Celebrations create opportunities for bonding. By sharing in their joys, we foster a sense of togetherness and connection that can be especially valuable as our relationships evolve.

- **Motivation:** Recognizing their achievements can serve as motivation for them to continue striving for their goals. It reinforces the idea that hard work and perseverance pay off.

Supporting Them Through Failure and Rejection

We all know that life is tough. Things don't always turn out the way we hope. So, how can we help our grown-up kids deal with failure and rejection?

Failure and rejection are an inevitable part of life, and our adult children are no exception. They will face setbacks in their careers, relationships, and personal pursuits. How we respond as parents can have a profound impact on their ability to cope and bounce back.

Case study: John, a 28-year-old, had applied for his dream graduate program but received a rejection letter. He was devastated and felt like he had let everyone down. As a parent, you can help in the following ways:

- **Active listening:** Listen without judgment. Sometimes, they just need someone to vent their frustrations to.
- **Empathy:** Offer empathy and let them know that it's okay to feel disappointed. Share your own experiences of rejection to show them that it's a universal part of life.
- **Encouragement:** Encourage them to learn from the experience. Failure can be a powerful teacher. Help them see the silver lining and how they can grow from it.
- **Respect their choices:** Respect their decisions on how to move forward. Sometimes, they may need time to reassess their goals or try a different path.

Coping strategies can play a significant role when our adult children are dealing with rejection and failure in life. These strategies can greatly impact how they navigate these difficult moments and ultimately influence their emotional well-being and resilience. As parents, understanding and supporting the coping strategies they employ is essential. Here's a reminder of some that may factor in:

Emotional Expression and Processing

- **Venting and talking:** Some adult children may choose to express their emotions openly by talking to friends, family, or a therapist. They seek comfort and support through conversation and sharing their feelings.

- **Journaling:** Writing in a journal can be a therapeutic way to process emotions and thoughts. Encourage them to explore their feelings through writing if they find it helpful.

Problem-Solving and Active Coping

- **Setting goals:** Encourage your adult children to set realistic goals and create a plan to address the situation that led to rejection or failure. This proactive approach can help them regain a sense of control.

- **Seeking feedback:** Some may choose to seek feedback from the rejection or failure to learn and improve. This constructive feedback can be valuable for personal growth.

Self-Care and Stress Reduction

- **Physical activity:** Regular exercise can be a powerful way to relieve stress and improve mood. Encourage them to engage in physical activities they enjoy.

- **Mindfulness and meditation:** Techniques like mindfulness and meditation can help manage anxiety and promote a sense of calm during difficult times.

Distraction and Avoidance

- **Engaging in hobbies:** Some may find solace in their hobbies and use them as a way to temporarily distract themselves from the emotional distress.
- **Avoidance:** While it's important to face challenges, there may be moments when they need a break from the stressor. This is okay as long as it doesn't become a long-term avoidance strategy.

Acceptance and Self-Compassion

Practicing self-compassion: Teach them the significance of showing kindness to themselves during challenging moments. Self-compassion entails treating oneself with the same kindness and understanding as one would extend to a dear friend.

Lastly, let's address a common concern: What if our adult children feel they have no purpose in life?

Helping Them Find Purpose

It's not uncommon for young adults to grapple with feelings of purposelessness. They may question their career choices, life goals, or even their existence. As parents, our role is to offer support and guidance. As parents, you can play a crucial role in helping your adult children develop adaptive coping strategies when they struggle with purposelessness or maladaptive behaviors. Here's how:

- **Talk to them:** Initiate conversations with your adult child about their coping mechanisms in a supportive and nonjudgmental manner. Foster a safe and open space for them to freely express their thoughts and feelings.

- **Role modeling:** Set an example by demonstrating healthy coping techniques in your own life. Show how you manage stress and challenges effectively.

- **Encourage self-awareness:** Help them identify the triggers that lead to their maladaptive coping strategies. Encouraging self-awareness can be the first step toward positive change.

- **Offer alternative solutions:** Collaborate with your child to brainstorm and develop a list of alternative coping strategies that they can try when faced with stress or difficult emotions.

- **Set boundaries:** If their maladaptive coping mechanisms are disruptive or harmful to themselves or others, establish clear boundaries and consequences. Make it known that such behaviors are not acceptable.

- **Educate:** Share information about healthy coping mechanisms and the long-term benefits of using them. Encourage them to explore alternatives to their maladaptive strategies.

Case study: Sarah, a 25-year-old, was struggling with a sense of purpose after being fired from a job she loved. Here's how you can assist:

- **Open dialogue:** Have open and nonjudgmental conversations about their feelings. Sometimes, just talking about their concerns can provide clarity.

- **Exploration:** Encourage them to explore new interests and hobbies. Often, purpose is found through experimentation.

- **Volunteering and giving back:** Suggest engaging in volunteer work or helping others. This can bring a sense of fulfillment and purpose.

- **Professional help:** If their feelings of hopelessness persist, it may be necessary to seek professional guidance.

Remember, it's normal for young adults to go through periods of doubt and self-discovery. Assure them that these feelings are temporary and that they won't always feel sad and defeated. Your love, patience, and support can make a world of difference during these challenging times. Let's jump into the next chapter, where we will cover how we, as parents, can accept partners and friends of our adult children.

Chapter 10: Connecting With Your Adult Child's Partners and Friends

In this chapter, we're going to dive into one of the most transformative aspects of our relationship with our adult children—their circle of friends and romantic partners. This is a pivotal juncture in our journey, and it's essential that we navigate it with empathy, understanding, and an open heart.

Our children are no longer the wide-eyed, impressionable kids who looked up to us for every answer. They're exploring the world, making their own choices, and building their own lives. And a significant part of that process involves forming connections with new people who may become integral to their lives.

As parents, we might have reservations, concerns, or even fears about the friends and partners our children choose. It's only natural to worry; after all, we've spent their entire lives protecting, guiding, and shaping their values. But now, it's time to embrace a new perspective.

We cannot expect to have the same level of control over our adult children's relationships as we did when they were young. Our role has shifted from being the directors of their lives to becoming trusted advisors and supporters. It's not about losing influence; it's about evolving our influence into something more profound.

Understanding Your Feelings

First, it's essential to acknowledge your feelings honestly. You may find yourself questioning the compatibility, values, or character of your child's partner or friends. While it's natural to be concerned for your child's well-being, it's important to separate your concerns from your personal biases.

Ask yourself, "Why don't I like this person?" Reflect on whether your feelings are based on valid concerns or preconceived notions. It's essential to self-reflect and be honest about any biases you might hold.

When you have concerns about the people in their life, you need to express them in a way that fosters understanding rather than conflict.

Consider having a private and respectful conversation with your child. Start by acknowledging their feelings and your love and concern for their well-being. Express your concerns without being judgmental or confrontational. Use "I" statements to emphasize your feelings and perspective. For example, say, "I'm worried about how this situation might affect you," rather than making accusatory statements.

Equally important is how you listen to your child. Give your child the space to share their perspective and feelings about their partner or friends without interrupting or immediately offering solutions. Sometimes, they might have insights or concerns you weren't aware of, and listening can help bridge the gap between your perspectives.

As parents, it's essential to remember that our adult children have the right to make their own decisions, including choosing their partners. While we can provide guidance and support, we must respect their autonomy. Attempting to control their choices can strain your relationship and push them away.

Try to find common ground or shared values with your child's partner or friends. This can be a bridge for better understanding and acceptance. Look for opportunities to connect, share experiences, or engage in activities together. Over time, these shared moments can help build a more positive relationship.

If you find that your feelings toward your child's partner continue to be a source of tension, consider seeking guidance from a therapist or counselor. A professional can assist you in managing intricate emotions and offer tactics to enhance your relationship with your child and their partner.

Remember, your child's happiness is paramount, and their choice of partner plays a significant role in their life satisfaction. While it may be challenging to accept someone you don't like, fostering an atmosphere of love, acceptance, and open communication can lead to a more harmonious relationship with your adult child and their partner.

Be mindful of your coping strategy when dealing with this issue. If you are struggling with the relationship between your adult child and their partner, you could be using empathy and understanding to navigate these concerns. Approach the situation with sensitivity, and keep your focus on maintaining a positive relationship with your child.

In the end, our goal as parents is to see our children thrive and be happy, and sometimes that means accepting the people they choose to have in their lives. By approaching this situation with empathy and understanding, we can continue to be a source of support and love for our adult children as they navigate the complexities of adulthood.

I Don't Like the Partner My Child Chose

Kathy's Story

The mother of two boys, her oldest wasn't one who dated often. When he moved away for university, she had a talk with him about women, and he told her his focus was his education. He wasn't wrong, and for the next five years, his nose was in a book. In his mid- 20s, he believed he had fallen in love for the first time.

Kathy was introduced to this woman and immediately got a bad vibe. She noticed that she would interrupt her son and finish his sentences. She would make fun of his small things, like his nose or his laugh. When Kathy would make mention of it, her son would reassure her that it was just "how she was." As time went on, she would notice other things. Her son financially supported this young woman. She wasn't working or going to school. When she asked, she was met with resistance and told it was none of her business.

Friends and other family members started to speak up, and this brought about talk of wedding dresses and buying a house. She was terrified for her son. Everything came crashing down around him quickly. She mentioned wanting to go home to visit family. Her son drove her; it was a ten-hour drive. As she exited the car, she said, "Mail me my things; I'm not coming back."

Kathy would find out later that he gave her over $10,000 of his savings and just how toxic she had been to him. She was emotionally abusive and left her son a shell of the man he was. It would take years of therapy to get him back on track, and she felt guilty for not chasing her off sooner.

As his mother, she had to sit back because he is an adult and let him travel this path. She was able to express how she felt and share her worries, but that was it. We can't live our lives for them. It is one of the most difficult parts of being a parent at this stage.

How to Handle This

What happens when one of our adult children dates someone we don't like? Maybe we find them controlling, toxic, or just annoying. How do we handle this? It's a situation that most of us will encounter at some point in our journey as parents of grown-up kids.

Start by having a heart-to-heart conversation with your child, expressing your concerns and feelings without judgment. Share your perspective calmly, emphasizing that you care about their happiness and well-being above all else. Remember, this isn't about winning an argument; it's about understanding and supporting your child's choices.

Once you've shared your thoughts, it's essential to respect your child's boundaries and decisions. Ultimately, they are the ones who need to navigate their relationship. Sometimes, when we push too hard against a partner, it can strain the relationship with our child. Trust that they will learn and grow from their experiences.

Keep in mind that first impressions can be misleading, and people can change. A partner you initially dislike may evolve into someone you respect and care for over time. Be patient and willing to give them a chance to prove themselves.

Concentrate on the qualities that truly matter in a partner, such as their kindness, respect for your child, and shared values. Sometimes, the things we dislike at first glance turn out to be superficial concerns in the grand scheme of a loving and supportive relationship.

If you believe there are significant issues or red flags in your child's relationship and they are not receptive to your concerns, consider suggesting professional help. A counselor or therapist can provide valuable guidance and facilitate communication between all parties involved.

If your adult child is not receptive to your concerns or professional help, it can be a challenging situation for a parent. In such cases, it's essential to focus on your own coping strategies, specifically setting boundaries and practicing self-care:

- **Setting boundaries:** It's vital that you establish clear boundaries between your child's choices and your own well-being. Recognize that you cannot control their decisions, and attempting to do so may harm your relationship. Set limits on how much emotional investment and involvement you have in their relationship issues.

- **Self-care:** Prioritize your own emotional and mental well-being. Continue to engage in activities that bring you joy and fulfillment. Spend time with friends and engage in hobbies or interests that help you maintain your own sense of identity and happiness.

If They Just Bother You

Not everyone will be to your liking. Sometimes, people just don't mesh well, and it might leave you questioning what others see in them. In such situations, it's likely best to leave it be. Your child might also feel that you're crossing the boundaries of a parent–adult child relationship.

One thing you can ask yourself is: How well do you really know this person? Have you ever had a sincere conversation with them? A 2018 study indicates that after having a conversation with another, people are often more liked than they perceive (**Boothby et al., 2018**).

Perhaps engaging in more conversations with your adult child's partner could improve your perception of them.

They're Controlling

Your sociable and approachable child might unexpectedly express the need to consult with a "so and so" before accepting your invitation to lunch. Alternatively, their preferences may have shifted to align with "whatever so-and-so wants to do." While you may perceive it clearly, your child may not recognize that their romantic interest is exerting control over them. Confronting them about this is unlikely to yield positive results.

Observing your child with a controlling partner can pose challenges. Frequently, individuals who are controlling are afraid of losing control and have a strong desire to exert influence over their surroundings. This inclination can also manifest in their personal relationships.

It could also indicate a potential for future abuse. Establishing open communication with your child about your concerns may be beneficial. If they feel comfortable talking with you, they may seek advice if needed in the future.

If You Suspect Abuse

Abuse can manifest in various ways, such as physical, verbal, emotional, sexual, and financial. At times, it may be quite subtle, with your child's partner displaying excessive jealousy, disrespect, or belittlement toward them.

Providing emotional support for your child may be beneficial. In such situations, emotional support can involve:

- Keep in mind that you can only help someone who wants to be helped.

- Refrain from judging, criticizing, or shaming your child.

- Continue to be supportive of their needs.

- Refrain from speaking negatively about their partner.

Remember, we are here to support our children, even when their choices differ from our own. Keep an open heart, and try to see the positive aspects of your child's partner. In my own experience, I've witnessed my child's partners grow and change, and my initial reservations have often proven to be unfounded.

Handling Holidays and Family Gatherings

The holiday season and family gatherings can be a wonderful time to reconnect and create lasting memories. However, when you find yourself at odds with your adult child's choice of partner, these occasions can become challenging to navigate. It's crucial to approach this delicate situation with love, understanding, and a commitment to maintaining family bonds. Here's how to handle holidays and family gatherings when you don't agree with your adult child's choice of partner.

Focus on Your Child's Happiness

Above all, remember that your child's happiness is what matters most. While you may have concerns about their partner, it's essential to support your child's choices and prioritize their well-being. Recognize that your child's partner may have qualities and attributes that you might not fully understand or appreciate.

Keep the Bigger Picture in Mind

During family gatherings, it's easy to get caught up in differences or tensions related to your child's partner. Try to keep the bigger picture in mind—the love and unity of your family. Remind yourself of the joy and togetherness these gatherings can bring and focus on the positive aspects of the occasion.

Maintain Open Communication

Maintain open and respectful communication with your adult child about your concerns. Express your feelings in a nonconfrontational manner, emphasizing your love for them and your desire to see them happy. Listen to their perspective and be willing to understand their point of view.

Set Boundaries for Conversations

While it's essential to communicate your concerns, it's equally important to set boundaries for conversations about your child's partner during family gatherings. Avoid heated debates or confrontations that can lead to tension and hurt feelings. Choose an appropriate time and place to discuss your concerns privately with your child, if necessary.

Find Common Ground

During family gatherings, strive to find common ground with your child's partner. Focus on shared interests, hobbies, or values that you might have in common. Engaging in pleasant conversations about neutral topics can help build bridges and foster a sense of connection.

Show Respect and Kindness

Regardless of your reservations, always treat your child's partner with respect and kindness during family gatherings. Small acts of kindness, like offering a warm greeting, can go a long way in creating a positive atmosphere. Remember, you don't have to agree with everything to be courteous and considerate.

Choose Your Battles Wisely

Not every disagreement or difference of opinion needs to be addressed during family gatherings. Choose your battles wisely, and prioritize maintaining a harmonious atmosphere. If you feel the need to address a significant concern, consider doing so privately and respectfully.

How to Handle the Hurt

We've all been there—our child introduces us to someone who, for one reason or another, doesn't sit well with us. It might be because they seem controlling, exhibit narcissistic traits, or we've heard rumors of infidelity. These situations can be incredibly tough to handle, but it's crucial that we approach them with empathy, understanding, and open communication. After all, our primary goal is to support our adult children and help them make the best choices for themselves.

Many parents find themselves in this situation, and it can be a complex and emotional journey. Let's explore how to deal with a partner choice we don't like, especially when we suspect our adult child is dating someone who exhibits toxic behavior.

Start by having an open and nonjudgmental conversation with your adult child. Share your concerns and observations calmly and without accusation. Use "I" statements to express how you feel, such as "I'm worried about how I've seen this relationship affect you.

In dealing with a partner choice you don't like, especially when you suspect your adult child is dating someone who exhibits toxic behavior, it can be helpful to explain your receiving love language of "quality time" to your child. Allowing them to understand that spending one-on-one time, enjoying a nice dinner together, or meeting up for coffee just to reconnect will go a very long way.

Real-life example: When Sarah's daughter started dating someone who seemed controlling, she shared her concerns with her. She didn't criticize her partner but instead focused on expressing her love and concern for her well-being. This approach helped Sarah feel more comfortable discussing her daughter's relationship with her.

Remember that your adult child is now an independent individual capable of making their own choices. While you may not agree with their choice of partner, it's essential to respect their autonomy and support their decisions. They may be aware of issues in the relationship that you aren't privy to.

If you suspect your child is in a relationship with a narcissist or someone who is controlling, educate yourself about these personality types and their behaviors. Understanding the dynamics at play can help you approach the situation with more empathy and knowledge.

Make sure your adult child knows that you're there for them, no matter what. Offer your support without conditions, and let them know that you'll be there to help if they ever need it. Sometimes, just knowing they have a safe space to turn to can make all the difference.

Case study: Richard's son, David, once dated someone who had a history of infidelity. He didn't push him away or criticize his choice. Instead, he offered a listening ear and a shoulder to lean on when he needed it. Eventually, he realized the relationship wasn't healthy and ended it on his terms.

Gently encourage your adult child to reflect on their relationship and how it makes them feel. Often, they may not see the red flags until they step back and evaluate things objectively.

Personal story: Sam's daughter, Ellie, took some time to reflect on her controlling partner's behavior and eventually decided that the relationship wasn't bringing her happiness. She realized that she deserved better and chose to move on.

Dealing with a partner choice we don't like in our adult children's lives can be incredibly challenging. However, by maintaining open communication, respecting their autonomy, educating ourselves, providing unwavering support, and encouraging self-reflection, we can help them navigate these tough situations. Remember, our role as parents evolves as our children grow, and our ultimate aim is to be a source of love and guidance in their lives, no matter the challenges they face.

Stay connected with your child, continue to nurture your relationship with them, and offer a safe space for them to confide in you. You are their parent, and your love is a guiding light in their journey. Join me in the next chapter as we explore the importance of self-care. Why it is essential that you take care of yourself.

Chapter 11:
Putting You First

Remember when you were on an airplane and the flight attendant instructed you to put on your oxygen mask before assisting others, even your own child? The reason for this seemingly counterintuitive advice is simple yet profound: You can't help anyone effectively if you're not taking care of yourself first. The same principle applies to your role as a parent of adult children.

This chapter will explore why it's not only okay but imperative for you to prioritize self-care in your life. We'll discuss the importance of nurturing your physical, emotional, and mental well-being. You'll learn practical strategies to create a healthy balance between your own needs and those of your adult children.

So, let's start by reminding ourselves that by taking care of our own well-being, we become better equipped to provide the love, support, and guidance our adult children need as they navigate their own paths in this different world. It's time to put on our oxygen masks first and embrace the wonderful adventure of parenting adults.

Why Self-Care Matters

You see, when we become parents, our lives revolve around our children. We put their needs before ours, sacrifice sleep for those late-night feedings, and dedicate our time to nurturing them. However, as they grow into adulthood, the dynamic shifts, and we find ourselves grappling with new challenges. It's easy to get caught up in the whirlwind of their lives, but remember, we deserve care and attention too.

Think of it this way: To be the best parent and maintain a healthy relationship with your adult children, you need to be in good shape mentally, emotionally, and physically. Self-care is not selfish; it's essential. Here's why:

- **Stress reduction:** Parenting, especially during times of transition or conflict, can be incredibly stressful. Engaging in self-care practices helps reduce stress levels, making you better equipped to handle challenges calmly.

- **Improved communication:** When you're well-rested and emotionally balanced, you communicate more effectively. This, in turn, fosters healthier discussions with your adult children.

- **Setting an example:** Demonstrating self-care teaches your children valuable life lessons. By prioritizing your well-being, you're showing them the importance of self-respect and self-love.

- **Enhanced emotional resilience:** Self-care builds emotional resilience, helping you bounce back from setbacks and cope with the inevitable ups and downs of life.

Types of Self-Care

Self-care is a personal journey, and what works for one person may not work for another. It's vital that you find practices that resonate with you. Here are some ideas:

- **Physical self-care:** Regular exercise, a balanced diet, adequate sleep, and annual health check-ups are fundamental components of physical self-care.

- **Emotional self-care:** Journaling, therapy, meditation, or mindfulness exercises can help you understand and manage your emotions better. There are some great apps for your phone or tablet for meditation and journaling to get you started.

- **Social self-care:** Maintaining relationships outside of your family is essential. Schedule time with friends, join clubs or groups of interest, or even consider volunteering. This gives you an opportunity to remind yourself of who you once were and who you want to become.

- **Intellectual self-care:** Stimulate your mind by reading, taking up a hobby, or enrolling in a course that interests you. Feed that brain and boost your cognitive power.

- **Spiritual self-care:** Explore your spiritual beliefs, whether through prayer, meditation, or simply spending time in nature. It is great for the soul.

But what if you feel guilty about taking time for yourself? Many parents find it challenging to deal with their own needs. It's important to remember that prioritizing self-care is not neglecting your children; it's nurturing your relationship with them. Here's how to deal with that guilt:

- **Reframe your perspective:** Realize that by caring for yourself, you're modeling self-respect and self-love, which your adult children can learn from and emulate.

- **Communicate:** Have an open and honest conversation with your children about your need for self-care. They may not only understand but also encourage it.

- **Set boundaries:** Establish boundaries that allow you to balance your own needs with your responsibilities toward your children.

- **Start small:** Begin with small self-care routines and gradually build them into your daily or weekly schedule. This can make the transition smoother and less guilt-inducing.

Remember, self-care isn't a luxury; it's a necessity. Just as our children's lives evolve, so must our approach to parenting them. By nurturing ourselves, we create a stronger foundation for the ever-changing relationship with our adult children.

Dealing With Feeling Unappreciated by Grown-Up Kids

One of the most common and painful emotions that parents of adult children experience is a sense of being unappreciated. You've poured your heart, soul, time, and energy into raising your children, and it's only natural to expect a little gratitude. However, life doesn't always work that way, and adult children may not always express their appreciation as readily as we'd like them to.

Remember, their lives are busy and filled with their own challenges. Sometimes, they may not even realize how much you've done for them. I want you to keep in mind their personality types as well. Some personality traits and tendencies may make it slightly more challenging for them to express gratitude to their parents. For example:

- **Introverted types (e.g., ISTJ, INTJ, INFJ, ISFJ):** Introverted individuals may find it somewhat challenging to express their emotions openly. They may internalize their gratitude and appreciation rather than openly expressing it.

- **Thinking types (e.g., INTJ, ISTP, ENTJ, ESTJ):** Thinking types tend to prioritize logical analysis and may not always be as comfortable expressing their emotions, including gratitude, as feeling types.

- **Perceiving types (e.g., INFP, ENTP, ESFP, ISTP):** Perceiving types may sometimes struggle with consistency in their expressions of gratitude, as they tend to be more adaptable and spontaneous.

The key here is communication. Don't be afraid to express your feelings in a nonconfrontational way. Share your thoughts, but also be open to hearing their perspective. It's important to foster an environment where they feel comfortable expressing their gratitude in their own way.

Dealing With a Controlling, Manipulative, or Guilt-Tripping Adult Child

Parenting doesn't come with a playbook, and sometimes we find ourselves in challenging situations. If you're dealing with an adult child who exhibits controlling, manipulative, or guilt-tripping behavior, it can be emotionally draining.

First, you need to set healthy boundaries. Remember, you are still their parent, and boundaries are a way to show love and respect for both parties. Calmly and assertively communicate your boundaries, and be consistent in enforcing them. Your health and feelings matter. Seek professional guidance if necessary to navigate these difficult situations.

Renee's Story

Renee is a single mom of three. Parenting has always been a struggle, but she has managed to maintain a decent relationship with all of her children. She allowed them the freedom to express their individuality. They knew she would always be there for them and love them, no matter what. Her middle child, Alexa, proved to be difficult. She was ungrateful and often appeared "spoiled" as a younger child.

As an adult, Alexa was demanding of her mother's time. She would show up with her two young children without notice and expect a babysitter. She would be gone for an entire weekend. She would demand money, rides to places, and constant favors. She never asked; she expected.

When Renee would try to have a discussion about this behavior, she was met with hostility and anger. She would tell her mother, "It's the least you can do; you are the reason I grew up without a father!" She would try to use guilt and manipulation to get what she wanted.

It would be Renee's two other children who would ultimately intervene in this situation. Giving their mother a voice and telling their sister that her behavior would no longer be tolerated, they emphasized that their mother deserved respect. They pointed out how they handle similar situations. If they would like their mother to babysit, they ask well in advance. If they need a favor, they offer one in return. They prioritize their mother's well-being above their conveniences.

Managing Guilt About Past Parenting Mistakes

We all make mistakes as parents; it's part of being human. Regret and guilt about past parenting decisions can haunt us, especially as our children become adults. It's important to recognize that you did your best with the knowledge and resources available to you at the time. If you are a parent who uses blame as a coping strategy, it can be helpful to do the following:

- Acknowledge self-blame and its negative impact on your well-being.
- Practice self-compassion, acknowledging that you did your best with what you knew.
- Accept imperfection as a natural part of parenting.
- Forgive yourself for past decisions, as holding onto guilt is counterproductive.

Christine's Story

Christine grew up with a toxic, narcissistic mother. She always hated hearing, "I did the best I could." Why? Because she didn't believe it. She felt this was a cop-out for her mom. She didn't realize this until she, herself, became a mom. Over the years, she would make mistakes of her own. We are human; this is expected. The difference between her and her mother? Her mistakes were never intentional, and she always took responsibility for them. She would sit her children down, explain the mistake, and discuss how she could have handled it differently. She would start with, "I did not do the best I could, and here is why." She would show her children accountability and a path to move forward. In later years, her adult children would tell her how much they always appreciated and respected this.

If you feel the need, apologize to your children for any mistakes you acknowledge. But remember, it's equally important to forgive yourself. Guilt can be a heavy burden, and carrying it into your relationship with your adult children won't benefit anyone. Seek support from a therapist or counselor if you find it challenging to let go of this guilt.

Dealing With Feelings of Resentment or Anger Toward Your Grown-Up Kids

Resentment and anger can surface when our adult children make choices that we disagree with or when they hurt us in some way. We need to acknowledge these feelings without judgment. It's okay to feel anger or resentment, but it's essential to find healthy ways to process and express these emotions.

Sit and have an honest, calm conversation with your child about your feelings, but also be willing to listen to their side of the story. Remember that their decisions are ultimately their own, and as adults, they have the right to make choices, even if they differ from what you'd hoped for them.

The biggest lesson to take away from this is that your feelings are valid. I know plenty of mothers who don't believe they are justified in feeling resentment because this is their child. Own your feelings and validate them, as this is what will help you process them. If we try to ignore them because we think we aren't supposed to feel them, we shove them down deep, leading to more resentment.

Parenting is about guiding and nurturing, but it's also about letting go.

You haven't failed as a parent if your child doesn't follow your advice or holds different beliefs. In fact, it's a sign of their independence and growth. Celebrate their individuality, and cherish the moments when you can offer support and guidance without judgment.

Don't allow society, friends, or family to make you feel differently if your child decides not to go to university and instead wants to travel. Don't allow others to feel less of your child if they want to explore the arts and not engineering. Far too often, parents get into a competitive state of mind and say, "Oh, my son is a blah blah, and my daughter does, yadda, yadda," as if their accomplishments are an extension of themselves. Yet, if that same child removed themselves from school to travel the world, it would be seen as "embarrassing" instead of a chance of a lifetime. We whisper in the shadows if our child wants to take a risk and open a business instead of becoming a dentist. If you keep this in mind, you may feel less agitated, upset, awkward, or offended if you suggest they spend five years in school and they announce they are joining a band.

Adjusting to Retirement and Parenting Adult Children

For some of us, retirement is on the horizon or already a reality. This transition can be challenging, especially when we're still actively parenting adult children. You might find yourself asking, "How do I balance my newfound freedom with my continued role as a parent?"

Realize that it's perfectly okay to enjoy your retirement and pursue your passions. You deserve it! Be available for your adult children when they require your support. Finding the right balance for you and your family is key. There are specific steps parents can take to help them navigate the transition into retirement while continuing to parent adult children. Here are some practical tips:

- **Communicate openly** about your retirement plans and expectations, emphasizing your desire for freedom while being available when needed.

- **Set boundaries** to balance your personal time with their independence, preventing misunderstandings.

- **Encourage their independence** while offering guidance, easing your parenting responsibilities.

- **Prioritize self-care** to maintain balance and be emotionally available when they seek support.
- **Collaborate on family matters** through open discussions and consensus-building.
- **Plan family time** for bonding and lasting memories.
- **Stay flexible** in adjusting your level of involvement based on changing circumstances.

Kyla and Ray's Story

Ray had long been dreaming of his retirement. He and his wife, Kyla, made plans to purchase an RV and travel far and wide. She could work remotely from the road, and he could do all the driving. They had been planning this dream for the last three years. As the time got closer, Kyla became more anxious. Despite their four children all being over the age of 25, she felt being away from them would be too hard. Worries about things going wrong and her not being immediately available kept her up at night.

Many long conversations with her husband, as he reassured her they instilled values and resilience in their children and they would be fine, didn't help. Three of her children were supportive, but the baby wasn't ready to let go of mom just yet.

That would all change when they started seriously dating. Mom leaving was no longer an issue. Ray chuckled and reminded his wife that, as he continually said, "Once they all get busy, it's just the two of us."

When They Move Far Away

One of the toughest moments in this journey can be when your adult child decides to move far away. It's completely natural to feel a sense of loss and loneliness when they're no longer just a short drive away.

Take a deep breath and remember that distance doesn't have to mean disconnection. Make use of technology to stay in touch. Set up regular video calls, exchange messages, and plan visits when possible. It might not be the same as having them close, but it can help make the distance seem less daunting.

Ah, the infamous empty nest syndrome. It's a real emotional rollercoaster, isn't it? When your last child leaves the nest, it's completely normal to feel a mix of emotions—sadness, loneliness, even a bit of relief.

The key is to acknowledge these feelings and give yourself permission to grieve the phase of life that's ending. But remember, this isn't the end of your story; it's the beginning of a new chapter. Use this time to rediscover your own interests and passions. Reconnect with your partner, if you have one, and focus on your own well-being.

One of the most challenging aspects of parenting adult children can be feeling left out of their lives. They're busy building their own paths, and sometimes it can feel like they're moving forward without you.

First, talk with them about how you feel. They might not even be aware of your feelings of exclusion. And remember, it's not a rejection of you; it's just the way life goes sometimes. Keep reinventing your relationship with them and yourself.

Coping Strategies for Loneliness

Loneliness can creep in when you're not actively involved in your children's day-to-day lives. To combat this, it's essential to invest in your own social connections and interests. Join clubs or groups that align with your hobbies. Rekindle old friendships or make new ones. The key is to create a life that's fulfilling and engaging beyond your role as a parent.

Lastly, let's acknowledge the emotional rollercoaster that comes with parenting adult children. It's a ride filled with highs and lows, joys and challenges. And that's perfectly okay. Embrace it all, knowing that it's a testament to the deep love you have for your children.

Your path will be unique, just as your relationship with your adult children is unique. The key is to stay open, communicate, and adapt as needed.

Remember, it's all part of the journey. We're here to learn and grow together, embracing the challenges and joys that come with parenting adult children. In the chapters ahead, we'll explore more ways to strengthen our relationships and create a loving, supportive environment for ourselves and our grown-up kids.

Chapter 12:
Your Adult Child Is Moving Back Home—Now What?

Ah, the nest—that cozy, warm place where we once nurtured our fledglings as they grew into the amazing adults we always knew they would become. But what happens when those very same adults decide to return to the nest or never leave it in the first place? Well, you've found your way to Chapter 12, and I'm here to guide you through this complex and often emotionally charged scenario.

This chapter is all about exploring the challenges and joys of having adult children back in the nest. We'll explore managing shared living spaces, fostering open communication, and setting healthy boundaries.

So, if you're currently navigating the complexities of having adult children living with you or contemplating what it would be like, you've come to the right place.

In the pages ahead, we'll explore practical strategies, share heartfelt stories, and most importantly, remind ourselves that change, growth, and adaptation are the cornerstones of parenting in the world today. Together, we'll uncover the tools and insights needed to make this journey as rewarding as it can be.

When Adult Children Stay at Home

Let's start by addressing the scenario where your adult child seems content to stay at home indefinitely, even when they should be branching out on their own. This situation can be disheartening, especially if you're providing financial support while they focus on sleeping or gaming all day. It's essential to approach this with love, understanding, and a good dose of realism.

Case Study: Sasha and David

Take Sarah and David, for instance. Sasha, a loving mother, noticed that her son David, who was about to graduate, showed no interest in moving out. He spent most of his time playing video games, and she continued to pay for his expenses. Sasha's concerns grew, and she couldn't understand why David didn't seem motivated to become independent.

First, it's important to understand that this situation is not uncommon in today's economic landscape. The transition to adulthood can be challenging, and factors such as high student loan debt, a competitive job market, and the rising cost of living can make it financially challenging for young adults to strike out on their own.

Start by having an open and nonjudgmental conversation with your adult child about their goals and aspirations. Ask them about their plans and how they envision their future. Avoid pushing them to leave, but express your concerns and set clear expectations regarding their responsibilities at home.

Establishing boundaries is vital. Discuss how you can gradually reduce financial support and encourage them to take on more responsibilities, such as paying rent or contributing to household expenses and duties. This not only helps your child develop financial independence but also reinforces the idea that they are responsible for their life choices.

Support their personal development by encouraging them to pursue hobbies, interests, or education that align with their goals. Help them explore opportunities for internships, part-time jobs, or volunteering to gain valuable experience and build a sense of purpose.

When Adult Children Change After Returning Home

Another common situation is when your adult child comes back home after college, but they seem like a different person. This can be challenging, as you may expect them to be the same as when they left.

Case Study: Emily and Michael

Consider Emily, who welcomed her son Michael back home after he finished college. She was surprised by the changes in his beliefs, interests, and lifestyle. Michael had adopted new habits and perspectives that didn't align with how she raised him, which left Emily feeling bewildered and concerned.

Adapting to Change

It's essential to remember that change is a natural part of growing up. Your adult child has been exposed to new experiences, ideas, and people, which can reshape their outlook on life. Instead of resisting these changes, try to embrace them as opportunities for growth. To view these changes as opportunities for growth, the parent of an adult child can

- maintain an open mind and embrace change for personal development.
- consider change as a chance to learn and broaden their perspective.
- enhance empathy by connecting with their adult child's experiences.
- embrace change to foster resilience and adaptability.

- strengthen their relationship by respecting their growth and autonomy.
- use change as an opportunity for personal growth and self-discovery.
- stay relevant by understanding new ideas and perspectives.
- embrace diversity and promote inclusivity in their family and community.
- encourage lifelong learning for everyone.
- lead by example, demonstrating a willingness to adapt and grow.

Ultimately, embracing change as an opportunity for growth is a mindset shift. By seeing change through a positive lens, you can navigate transitions within your family with resilience, empathy, and a commitment to personal and collective development.

Here are some steps you can take to help you adapt to these changes:

Open dialogue: Initiate conversations with your child about their experiences and the changes they've undergone. Seek to understand their perspective and the reasons behind their transformation. This can lead to greater empathy and strengthen your bond.

Respect their autonomy: Recognize that your adult child is an independent individual with their own values and beliefs. While you may not agree with everything they do or believe in, respecting their autonomy is important for maintaining a healthy relationship. Try to reflect on yourself at this age. Did your parents always agree with your choices? Did you wish they had been more supportive?

Common ground: Discover mutual interests and common ground to bridge the gap between your expectations and their evolving identity. This has the potential to foster meaningful connections and mutual understanding.

Remember that your relationship with your adult child is evolving, and adapting to these changes is part of the journey. While it may not be the same as when they were children, it can be equally rewarding and fulfilling in its own way.

The Nest Is Full Again

When our adult children decide to move back in, it can be a challenging scenario, but by setting clear expectations, contributions, and house rules, we can create a harmonious living arrangement that respects everyone's needs and desires.

Setting expectations, contributions, and house rules:

- **Agree on a timeline and action plan:** One of the first steps when your adult child decides to move back in or never leaves is to sit down and have an open and honest conversation. Instead of making unilateral decisions, involve your child in setting a timeline and creating an action plan. This approach allows them to have a say in their own future, promoting a sense of responsibility and cooperation.
    - **Real-life example:** Gerry's son, Jack, moved back in after he lost his job. We discussed his goals, his expected length of stay, and how he could contribute financially. We agreed that he would stay for a year while saving money for his own place. This gave him a clear purpose and a sense of direction. Jack, being an INTJ (Introverted Intuition, Thinking, Judging) personality type, appreciated this because he is a strategic thinker who likes to plan and set long-term goals.
- **Giving space and respecting privacy:** As our children become adults, they crave independence and privacy. It's essential to respect their boundaries while balancing the dynamics of a shared living space. Acknowledge that your adult

child is no longer a teenager and deserves privacy and personal space.

- **Real-life example:** When my daughter, Sam, moved back home temporarily, we designated certain areas of the house as her private space. We also communicated about her schedule and when she might need alone time. This helped us avoid unnecessary conflicts and promote a sense of harmony in our home. Sam appreciated this because, as an (I) Introvert personality type, she truly values her personal space. She finds alone time necessary to recharge her batteries.

- **Contributions and responsibilities:** Encourage your adult child to contribute to the household in a way that is fair and reasonable. This can include sharing the cost of utilities, groceries, or rent, depending on their financial situation. Having responsibilities can make them feel like a valuable part of the household.

    - **Real-life example:** When Connor's son Jack moved back in. We agreed that he would contribute to groceries and help with chores. This not only lightened our load but also helped him feel like he was contributing to the family.

- **House rules:** Establish clear house rules that everyone agrees upon. These rules should cover important aspects like quiet hours, cleaning responsibilities, and shared spaces. Having these boundaries in place can prevent misunderstandings and conflicts.

    - **Real-life example:** The Cosgrove's had a family meeting to create a list of house rules that applied to everyone. These rules included keeping noise levels down after 10 p.m. and ensuring that shared spaces, like the kitchen, were kept clean. This way, they all had a clear understanding of what was expected. This helped their daughter Alexa because she is an ESTJ (Extraverted Sensing, Thinking, Judging) personality type. She is practical and results-oriented. She appreciates rules that help her achieve her results efficiently.

Don't Fall Into the Enabling Trap

There are those of us parents who love the idea of our adult children moving back home. We have missed them ever since they left. We can find ourselves making their stay quite comfortable, making their favorite meals, redecorating a room, and well, enabling them.

Addressing separation anxiety and enabling behavior, whether from a parent or your partner, requires awareness, empathy, and open communication. Here's how a parent or partner can navigate this situation:

Parent with separation anxiety:

- **Self-reflection:** Reflect on your feelings and actions. Acknowledge any anxiety or discomfort you may have about your adult child living independently. Understanding your emotions is the first step.

- **Establish boundaries:** If your adult child has moved back home and your behavior is enabling their dependency, set clear boundaries. Communicate your expectations for their independence and responsibilities while living with you.

- **Encourage independence:** Support your adult child in their pursuit of independence. Help them set goals and make plans for the future. Encourage them to take steps toward self-sufficiency.

- **Open communication:** Have a gentle and understanding conversation with your child about your feelings and concerns. Express your love and support while explaining the importance of their independence.

Partner enabling the behavior:

- **Choose the right time:** Find a suitable moment to discuss the enabling behavior with your partner. Avoid bringing it up during a heated argument or when emotions are high.

- **Use "I" statements:** Frame your concerns using "I" statements to avoid sounding accusatory. For example, say, "I feel concerned about our adult child's dependency, and I believe it's affecting their growth."

- **Express empathy:** Show empathy toward your partner's perspective and feelings. Acknowledge that they may be acting out of love and concern for your child. Keep in mind that their receiving love language may be quality time or acts of service.

- **Share the impact:** Explain how enabling behavior can hinder your adult child's development and independence. Share specific examples of situations where this behavior has had negative consequences.

- **Offer solutions together:** Instead of criticizing, propose solutions as a team. Suggest ways both of you can support your child's growth and independence while maintaining a loving environment.

- **Set boundaries together:** Work together to establish clear boundaries and expectations for your adult child. This can help both you and your partner align on your parenting approach.

- **Prioritize your relationship:** Ensure that your concerns about enabling behavior don't strain your relationship with your partner. Reaffirm your commitment to each other and your shared values.

Addressing enabling behavior and separation anxiety is a sensitive matter that requires patience and understanding. The key is to approach the situation with empathy, focusing on the well-being and independence of your adult child while maintaining a healthy relationship with your partner.

Navigating the transition when your adult child either never leaves or moves back in can be challenging, but with constant communication, mutual respect, and clear boundaries, it's possible to maintain a harmonious and supportive living arrangement. Remember, we are all evolving in this changing world, and our relationships with our adult children require the same adaptability and love that we've provided since their first steps. It is time to move into our last chapter, where we will discuss the best ways to support our adult children through the toughest times in life.

Chapter 13:
How You Can Support Your Adult Child Through Difficult Situations

Life's journey is not always smooth, and our children, despite their growth and independence, will inevitably face major life events and challenges. Whether it's pursuing a new career, navigating a relationship, dealing with health issues, or just figuring out this maze called adulthood, they'll need our guidance, understanding, and unwavering support.

We can't erase the challenges or life events our adult children will encounter, but we can be a sturdy anchor in the storm, a shoulder to lean on, and a source of unwavering love and encouragement. So, let's explore this chapter together and ensure that our children always know they have a loving and supportive parent by their side, ready to help them weather life's storms.

Navigating Major Life Transitions

Life is a series of transitions. From the moment our children are born, we guide them through countless milestones—the first day of school, learning to ride a bike, getting a driver's license, and so much more. But what happens when those milestones transition into something even more complex: adulthood?

Marriage: Embrace Their Choices

One of the most significant milestones your adult child may encounter is marriage. It's important to remember that they are forming their own family unit, and this can be an exciting yet challenging time for everyone involved.

- **Avoid interfering:** While your parental instincts may kick in, it's crucial to respect their choices. Whether they are marrying for love, companionship, or even convenience, offer your support without judgment. If you have concerns, communicate them calmly and without pressure.

- **Maintain boundaries:** Understand that their priorities may shift, and their partner will play a significant role in their life. It's okay to set boundaries, but do so with love and respect, allowing them space to build their relationship.

- **Financial expectations:** Discuss openly any financial considerations surrounding the marriage. Does your adult child need help with wedding expenses? Do you, as the parents, want to assist with a portion of these expenses? Have you discussed helping with the down payment of their first home? Will the newlywed couple need to stay with you while they save for a home of their own? While having these conversations, be mindful of everyone's personality styles and love languages. This can help us better understand the needs and motivations of all involved.

- **Celebrate their journey:** Share in their happiness and joy. Celebrate their milestones and cherish the moments when they include you in their life as a married couple.

Divorce: Be Their Rock

Divorce is a difficult transition for anyone, and when your adult child goes through it, your support can make a world of difference.

- **Listen without judgment:** When they confide in you, listen with an open heart. Avoid blaming or criticizing their decisions. They need empathy and a safe space to share their feelings.

- **Offer practical help:** Be there to help with logistics, childcare, or emotional support, depending on their needs. Sometimes, practical assistance can ease their burden during this challenging time.

- **Encourage healing:** Encourage them to seek professional help if necessary, such as therapy or counseling. Your role is to support their well-being, even if it means seeking help outside of your abilities. It is important to remind yourself of their coping strategies during this time. For example, if your child uses diversion and distraction, you could suggest engaging in activities that provide a temporary diversion from the stress of the divorce, such as watching a movie together, going for a hike, or pursuing a creative hobby.

Parenthood: Respect Their Choices

When your child becomes a parent, your role as a grandparent can be both rewarding and complicated. Remember that they are the parents now, and your role is to support, not dictate.

- **Respect parenting choices:** Understand that their parenting style may differ from yours. Offer advice when asked, but avoid unsolicited criticism. Trust that they will make the best choices for their child. This should never be an issue of "I raised you, so I know better." This is not your child, so making decisions without consulting the parents is unacceptable.

- **Be available but not intrusive:** Offer to babysit or help when they need a break, but respect their boundaries as parents. Remember, they are learning just as you did when you became a parent.

- **Enjoy this role:** Be mindful of what the role of a grandparent means. This is not a time for a "do over" if you feel you made mistakes as a parent. This child shouldn't have to be responsible for any past issues. Love and enjoy them for who they are.

- **Celebrate grandparenting:** Cherish the special moments you have with your grandchildren. Your experience can be a valuable resource, but let your adult child take the lead in their parenting journey.

Career Changes: Encourage Growth

Career transitions can be exciting or daunting for your adult children. Your support and guidance can help them navigate these changes successfully.

- **Celebrate their ambitions:** Encourage their career aspirations and celebrate their achievements, whether it's a new job, a career shift, or entrepreneurial ventures.

- **Offer guidance, not pressure:** Share your experiences and knowledge, but avoid pushing them into a career path they don't want. Let them make their own decisions.

- **Provide a safety net:** In times of career uncertainty, be their safety net—emotionally and, if possible, financially. This can provide the security they need to take calculated risks.

Job Loss

Harrison's son, Mark, who was a successful IT professional, found himself out of a job due to the company downsizing. It was a shock to him, and he felt overwhelmed by the uncertainty of the future. In that moment, Harrison had to put his parenting skills to the test in a different way:

- **Talk:** The first thing Harrison did was to reach out and offer an open ear. He didn't jump into giving advice or solutions right away. Instead, he asked Mark how he felt and what he needed from him. This open communication allowed him to express his emotions without judgment.

- **Emotional support:** Job loss can be a blow to self-esteem and mental health. His dad made sure to reassure Mark that his worth was not tied to his job. They explored his interests and passions, focusing on building his self-confidence during this difficult period.

- **Respect boundaries:** It's essential to respect our children's boundaries as they navigate this challenging time, yet still encourage forward progress. Harrison didn't push Mark to share more than he was comfortable with, and he let him take the lead in seeking help when he was ready. In this case, if Mark engages in self-distraction or denial coping strategies, Harrison would approach the situation with empathy, support, and understanding. He could

    - express to his son that he needs to resume his job search.

    - have a respectful conversation in order to get the point across.

    - share resources for coping (therapy, support groups, etc.).

    - offer to help update his resume.

    - encourage his child to take ownership of their job search.

    - suggest attending industry-related events, workshops, or connecting with mentors or friends who can provide valuable insights and opportunities.

- **Encourage resilience:** While it's natural to want to shield our children from hardships, it's equally important to encourage resilience. Harrison and Mark discussed strategies for job hunting, including updating his resume, networking, and exploring new opportunities. Harrison also encouraged him to seek professional career counseling.

- **Stay positive:** Maintaining a positive outlook can be infectious. Harrison shared stories of people who had bounced back from job losses, emphasizing that setbacks often lead to growth and new opportunities.

Addiction Recovery

If you're reading this, you're likely facing one of the most challenging situations a parent can encounter—supporting an adult child through addiction recovery.

Addiction is a complex issue that can strike anyone, regardless of their background, upbringing, or the love we've poured into them throughout their lives. It's a battle that tests our patience, resilience, and the very essence of parenthood. It's a situation where the rules of parenting you once knew may no longer apply, and adapting to the times becomes crucial.

Let me start by saying this: Your child's struggle with addiction is not a reflection of your parenting. Addiction is a disease, and your child needs your support more than ever. In this chapter, we'll discuss how to provide that support effectively while maintaining healthy boundaries.

Understanding the Addiction

The first step is to educate yourself about addiction. Knowledge is your best ally in this battle. Attend support groups, read books, and consult experts to better understand the nature of addiction. This will help you empathize with your child's struggle and reduce the stigma often associated with it.

Keep Talking

Open and nonjudgmental communication is vital. Initiate conversations where your child feels safe sharing their feelings and experiences. Avoid blame and criticism, as they are counterproductive. Listen more than you speak, and acknowledge their pain.

Remember, our relationship with our adult children should evolve. It's no longer about giving orders or controlling their lives. It's about being a trusted confidant and a source of support.

Get Assistance From a Professional

Don't hesitate to seek professional guidance. Addiction recovery often requires a multifaceted approach involving therapists, doctors, and support groups. Encourage your child to seek help, and be there to assist them in finding suitable resources.

Establishing Limits

Support doesn't mean enabling destructive behavior. You need to set clear boundaries. For example, you can support your child emotionally, but you shouldn't financially support their addiction. Tough love can be a necessary, albeit painful, step.

Self-Care for Parents

Supporting a child through addiction recovery can be emotionally draining. Remember to take care of yourself. Seek therapy or counseling for yourself if needed. Prioritizing your mental and emotional well-being is not selfish; it's essential.

Let me share a personal story. My own son, John, battled addiction in his late twenties. It was heart-wrenching to watch him struggle, but through education, open communication, and professional assistance, we managed to support him as he traveled his journey to recovery. Today, he's a thriving, healthy adult.

I also want to introduce you to Lena, a friend of mine. She faced a similar situation with her daughter and found solace in local support groups. These communities provided a safe space for her to share her feelings and connect with others who understood her pain.

Research shows that parental support can play a pivotal role in addiction recovery. It helps them feel less isolated and more motivated to overcome their addiction. Studies emphasize the importance of a nonjudgmental, safe, and empathetic approach (**Hogue et al., 2021**).

Helping an adult child through addiction recovery demands a careful mix of empathy, boundaries, and professional assistance. As parents, our responsibilities may evolve, but our love and support are unwavering.

Understanding the Impact of Divorce on Your Grown-Up Kids

Let's start by acknowledging that divorce is a reality many families face. Whether it's your own divorce or that of your adult child, it can have a profound impact. But remember, it's not about blame; it's about understanding and support.

Adult children of divorce may react differently based on their personality types when it comes to their parents' new relationships and the impact of divorce on their own perceptions of long-term relationships:

- **ISTJ (The Inspector):** These individuals might approach their parents' new romance cautiously. They value stability and may feel uncomfortable with the uncertainty of a new relationship. They may also worry about how the divorce could affect their own commitment to long-term relationships.

- **ENFP (The Champion):** ENFPs may be more open to their parents' new romantic endeavors. They tend to be adaptable and might see this change as an opportunity for personal growth. However, they may still grapple with the emotional challenges that come with divorce.

- **INTP (The Thinker):** INTPs are analytical and may analyze the situation from a logical standpoint. They may question the reasons behind their parents' divorces and how it impacts their own beliefs about long-term relationships. They may need time to process their emotions.

It's important to recognize that each adult child will react uniquely to their parents' divorce and new relationships. Understanding their personality traits can offer insights into their reactions, but providing support, empathy, and understanding will go a long way.

Understanding Mental Health

Our children's mental health is paramount, and as parents, we have a vital role to play in supporting them through their struggles. Remember, it's not about fixing their problems; it's about being there for them, just as we've always been.

Older parents, particularly those in the boomer generation, may have certain misconceptions or make common mistakes when it comes to mental health. These can include:

- **Stigma:** Many older generations grew up in an era where mental health issues were often stigmatized and not openly discussed. As a result, they may view seeking help for mental health concerns as a sign of weakness or a lack of personal strength.

- **Minimization:** Some older parents may downplay the significance of mental health challenges, believing that previous generations faced adversity without the need for professional help. They may dismiss their children's struggles as "just a phase" or as something that will naturally pass.

- **Self-reliance:** The boomer generation often values self-reliance and independence. They may encourage their children to "tough it out" or handle their problems on their own, not fully understanding the benefits of seeking therapy or counseling.

- **Lack of awareness:** Some older parents may simply be unaware of the prevalence and impact of mental health issues in today's society. They may not recognize the signs or understand the importance of early intervention and treatment.

Before we dive into strategies, it's important to educate ourselves about mental health issues. Talk to experts, read books, and perhaps attend support groups. Understanding what your child is going through can help you approach the situation with empathy and knowledge.

Be sure to create an environment where your adult child feels safe discussing their feelings. Encourage conversations in a safe and loving environment. Start with, "I'm here to listen. How can I support you?" Sharing your own experiences can also help them feel less alone.

It is important to remember that our adult children are no longer kids. They have their own thoughts, feelings, and decisions to make. Respect their autonomy. Offer guidance, but let them ultimately decide their path.

If your adult child is struggling with depression or anxiety, suggest professional help. Offer to assist in finding a therapist or counselor who specializes in their specific needs. You can offer to go with them, drive them, or be there in any capacity they may need. Remember, therapy isn't a sign of weakness; it's a powerful tool for growth and healing.

Supporting someone with mental health issues is not a one-time effort; it's an ongoing journey. Be patient, even when progress seems slow or setbacks occur. Remind your child that you're there for the long haul.

While being supportive is vital, it's also essential to maintain boundaries. Sometimes, our adult children may lean on us excessively, which can become emotionally draining. Kindly communicate your boundaries while reassuring them of your love and support.

Mental health issues are complex and often arise from a combination of factors. We want to avoid stigmatizing language or attitudes; instead, foster an atmosphere of acceptance and understanding.

Let me share the story of my daughter, who faced severe anxiety during her college years. It would be well into her second year before she confided in me. She suffered through panic attacks and avoided class all together for all that time. She felt shame and embarrassment. My heart broke thinking she felt she couldn't come to me. I immediately reassured her that I too suffered from anxiety. I told her that I had been in therapy for a good part of my adult life and that I revisit it whenever I feel I need a tune-up. She started therapy, and I supported her by attending some sessions together. It wasn't always easy, but our commitment to her well-being helped her regain her confidence and overcome her anxiety.

Supporting adult children with mental health challenges is undoubtedly a delicate balancing act. It requires understanding, patience, and a willingness to adapt to their unique needs. Remember, you're not alone on this journey. Reach out to support groups or seek advice from other parents who've been through similar experiences. Together, we can create a loving and empathetic environment that helps our children thrive, even in the face of difficult life struggles.

Conclusion

As we come to the end of this journey together, I want to extend my heartfelt gratitude for taking the time to explore the pages of this book. We've embarked on a profound and transformative exploration of parenthood in the realm of adulthood, and I hope you've found it as enlightening and empowering as I intended it to be.

Throughout this book, we've tackled a myriad of topics, from communication and navigating transitions to the profound pain of estrangement. We've shared each other's stories, learned from experts, and dived deep into the realms of personality types, coping strategies, and love languages. Why? Because understanding these facets of our adult children empowers us to respond to them with compassion and wisdom.

In every word I've written, my aim has been to offer hope, empathy, understanding, and a sense of empowerment. To give parents an understanding of their child's perspective and help them change their own in the process. I've stressed the importance of growth and change, not only for our adult children but for us as parents as well. It's challenging to watch our beloved offspring venture out into the world and to see them stumble and hurt. But it's through these experiences that they learn and grow, and it's through our unwavering support that they find their way.

I encourage you to view this book as a trusted guide, one you can revisit whenever you need guidance or a reminder that you're not alone on this journey. Whether your child moves back in, starts their own family, or faces other life-altering transitions, these pages are here to provide insights and strategies to navigate these changes successfully.

As a mother of two adult children, I understand that this transition isn't easy. It's filled with uncertainty, joy, frustration, and fulfillment. But I also know, without a shadow of a doubt, that it is a worthwhile one. It's an evolution of our relationship with our children, a journey of discovery, and a testament to our enduring love for them.

Now, I'd like to ask for a small favor. If you found this book helpful, insightful, supportive, or empowering in any way, please consider leaving a review. Your review can help get this book into the hands of other parents who may be navigating the same challenging path, providing them with the guidance and support they need.

Thank you once again for sharing in this journey with me. May your relationship with your adult children continue to flourish, deepen, and bring you endless joy.

With warmest regards,

Belinda

If you enjoyed reading this book, please share your review by clicking this link:

https://bit.ly/parentadultchildrenreview

Or scan this QR code to leave your review:

References

Aikaterini Vasiou, Kassis, W., Αναστασία Κρασανάκη, Aksoy, D., Favre, C. A., & Spyridon Tantaros. (2023). Exploring parenting styles patterns and children's socio-emotional skills. *Children (Basel)*, *10*(7), 1126–1126. https://doi.org/10.3390/children10071126

Bailey, A. (2022, May 18). *Coping mechanisms: Everything you need to know.* Verywell Health. https://www.verywellhealth.com/coping-mechanisms-5272135

Barowski, J. (2023, November 21). *Maladaptive coping mechanisms and behavior.* Study.com. https://study.com/learn/lesson/maladaptive-coping-mechanisms-list-examples.html#:~:text=Examples%20of%20maladaptive%20coping%20strategies

Barrie, C., Bartkowski, J., & Haverda, T. (2019). The digital divide among parents and their emerging adult children: Intergenerational accounts of technologically assisted family communication. *Social Sciences*, *8*(3), 83. https://doi.org/10.3390/socsci8030083

Boothby, E. J., Cooney, G., Sandstrom, G. M., & Clark, M. S. (2018). The liking gap in conversations: Do people like us more than we think? *Psychological Science*, *29*(11), 1742–1756. https://doi.org/10.1177/0956797618783714

Borresen, K. (2024, January 11). *These 6 habits will transform your relationship with your adult kids.* HuffPost. https://www.huffpost.com/entry/better-relationship-adult-children-parent_l_651c3cdfe4b0b443172fd98e

Chapman, G. D. (2010). *The five love languages : How to express heartfelt commitment to your mate.* Manjul Pub.

Coping & stress management skills test. (n.d.). Psychology Today. https://www.psychologytoday.com/ca/tests/career/coping-stress-management-skills-test

Daniel, B. (2024, February 8). *Family estrangement: 6 ways to reconcile with adult children.* Focus on the Family. https://www.focusonthefamily.com/parenting/family-estrangement-6-ways-to-reconcile-with-adult-children/

Fletcher, J. (2021, August 31). *How to deal when you don't approve of your adult kid's relationship.* PsychCentral. https://psychcentral.com/lib/when-you-dont-approve-of-your-adult-childs-relationship

Halpert, J. (2022, September 6). *There is no road map for the longest phase of parenthood.* The Atlantic. https://www.theatlantic.com/family/archive/2022/09/parenting-advice-adult-children/671304/

Hendriksen, E. (2019, March 18). *Failure to launch syndrome.* Quick and Dirty Tips. https://www.quickanddirtytips.com/articles/failure-to-launch-syndrome/

Hogue, A., Becker, S. J., Wenzel, K., Henderson, C. E., Bobek, M., Levy, S., & Fishman, M. (2021). Family involvement in treatment and recovery for substance use disorders among transition-age youth: Research bedrocks and opportunities. *Journal of Substance Abuse Treatment, 129,* 108402. https://doi.org/10.1016/j.jsat.2021.108402

Karantzas, G. (2023, March 3). *Is there science behind the five love languages?* Greater Good. https://greatergood.berkeley.edu/article/item/is_there_science

_behind_the_five_love_languages#:~:text=According%20to%20Chapman%2C%20people%20are

Kaufman, G. (2013). *Necessary conversations.* Good Books.

Keep having conversations with adult children. (2016, December). HealthLink BC. https://www.healthlinkbc.ca/mental-health-substance-use/substance-use/parenting-and-substance-use/keep-having-conversations#:~:text=Showing%20your%20support%20and%20your

Kindelan, K. (2023, October 24). *Young adults twice as likely as teens to suffer from anxiety and depression, study finds.* ABC News. https://abcnews.go.com/GMA/Wellness/young-adults-teens-suffer-anxiety-depression-study-finds/story?id=104247559

Jill. (2021, February 22). *What to do when adult children won't leave home.* Living on a Dime. https://www.livingonadime.com/adult-child-wont-leave-home/

Ma, X., Yue, Z.-Q., Gong, Z.-Q., Zhang, H., Duan, N.-Y., Shi, Y.-T., Wei, G.-X., & Li, Y.-F. (2017). The effect of diaphragmatic breathing on attention, negative affect and stress in healthy adults. *Frontiers in Psychology*, *8*(874), 1–12. https://doi.org/10.3389/fpsyg.2017.00874

Mental Health Foundation. (2022). *How to look after your mental health using exercise.* https://www.mentalhealth.org.uk/explore-mental-health/publications/how-look-after-your-mental-health-using-exercise#:~:text=Studies%20show%20that%20there%20is

Myers-Briggs overview. (2023). Myers & Briggs Foundation. https://www.myersbriggs.org/my-mbti-personality-type/myers-briggs-overview/

Next Step 4 ADHD. (2020, December 14). *5 criteria for positive parenting with Dr. Jane Nelsen.* Next Step 4 ADHD.

https://nextstep4adhd.com/5-criteria-for-positive-parenting-with-dr-jane-nelsen/

Nguyen, J. (2020, October 21). *What are the 5 love languages? Everything you need to know.* Mindbodygreen. https://www.mindbodygreen.com/articles/the-5-love-languages-explained

Paramesti, M. (2022, May 9). *Do you know that celebrating your child's success matters for their future.* Beach Momz Child Development Center. https://www.beachmomz.com/do-you-know-that-celebrating-your-child-s-success-matters-for-their-future

Personality types. (2023). 16 Personalities. https://www.16personalities.com/personality-types

Sánchez-Núñez, M. T., García-Rubio, N., Fernández-Berrocal, P., & Latorre, J. M. (2020). Emotional intelligence and mental health in the family: The influence of emotional intelligence perceived by parents and children. *International Journal of Environmental Research and Public Health, 17*(17), 6255. https://doi.org/10.3390/ijerph17176255

Schofield, T. J., Conger, R. D., Donnellan, M. B., Jochem, R., Widaman, K. F., & Conger, K. J. (2012). Parent personality and positive parenting as predictors of positive adolescent personality development over time. *Merrill-Palmer Quarterly, 58*(2), 255–283. https://doi.org/10.1353/mpq.2012.0008

Seitzer, M. (2022, August 22). *Adult children | the guide to parenting adult children.* Extra Mile. https://extramile.thehartford.com/family/parenting/parenting-adult-children/

Sharpe, R. (2023, October 19). *14 coping mechanisms you can use for different situations.* Declutter the Mind. https://declutterthemind.com/blog/coping-mechanisms/

Sockle, B. (2023, February 22). *5 problems adult children of divorce face.* Divorce Lawyers for Men. https://www.divorcelawyersformen.com/blog/adult-children-of-divorce/#:~:text=Many%20adult%20children%20of%20divorce

Travers, M. (2023, April 27). *2 ways to get better at admitting when you're wrong.* Psychology Today. https://www.psychologytoday.com/intl/blog/social-instincts/202304/2-ways-to-get-better-at-admitting-when-youre-wrong

Why celebrating successes is important to our mental health. (2021, August 11). Innovative Resources. https://innovativeresources.org/why-celebrating-successes-is-important-to-our-mental-health/

Made in the USA
Middletown, DE
08 February 2026

28264237R00102